Precision Medicine

A Guide to Genomics in Clinical Practice

D1609576

Precision Medicine
A Guide to Genomics in Clinical Practice

Jeanette J. McCarthy, MPH, PhD
Adjunct Associate Professor
Community and Family Medicine and
Center for Applied Genomics and Precision Medicine
Duke University
Durham, North Carolina
Adjunct Associate Professor
Department of Medicine
University of California, San Francisco
San Francisco, California

Bryce A. Mendelsohn, MD, PhD
Assistant Clinical Professor
Department of Pediatrics, Division of Medical Genetics
University of California, San Francisco
UCSF Benioff Children's Hospitals
San Francisco, California

New York   Chicago   San Francisco   Athens   London   Madrid   Mexico City   Milan
New Delhi   Singapore   Sydney   Toronto

Precision Medicine: A Guide to Genomics in Clinical Practice

1 2 3 4 5 6 7 8 9   DSS   21 20 19 18 17 16

ISBN 978-1-259-64413-9
MHID 1-259-64413-8

Notice

Medicine is an ever-changing science. As new research and clinical experience broaden our knowledge, changes in treatment and drug therapy are required. The authors and the publisher of this work have checked with sources believed to be reliable in their efforts to provide information that is complete and generally in accord with the standards accepted at the time of publication. However, in view of the possibility of human error or changes in medical sciences, neither the authors nor the publisher nor any other party who has been involved in the preparation or publication of this work warrants that the information contained herein is in every respect accurate or complete, and they disclaim all responsibility for any errors or omissions or for the results obtained from use of the information contained in this work. Readers are encouraged to confirm the information contained herein with other sources. For example and in particular, readers are advised to check the product information sheet included in the package of each drug they plan to administer to be certain that the information contained in this work is accurate and that changes have not been made in the recommended dose or in the contraindications for administration. This recommendation is of particular importance in connection with new or infrequently used drugs.

This book was set in Minion by MPS Limited.
The editors were Amanda Fielding and Christina M. Thomas.
The production supervisor was Rick Ruzycka.
Project management was provided by Shubham Dixit, MPS Limited.
The cover designer was Dreamit, Inc.
RR Donnelley Shenzhen was printer and binder.

This book is printed on acid-free paper.

Library of Congress Cataloging-in-Publication Data

Names: McCarthy, Jeanette (Genetic epidemiologist), author. | Mendelsohn, Bryce, author.
Title: Precision medicine : a guide to genomics in clinical practice / Jeanette McCarthy, Bryce Mendelsohn.
Description: New York : McGraw-Hill Education, [2017] | Includes bibliographical references and index.
Identifiers: LCCN 2016021548| ISBN 9781259644139 (pbk. : alk. paper) | ISBN 1259644138
Subjects: | MESH: Genetic Testing | Genetic Predisposition to Disease | Precision Medicine | Genetics, Medical—ethics
Classification: LCC RB155 | NLM QZ 52 | DDC 616/.042—dc23 LC record available at https://lccn.loc.gov/2016021548

Contents

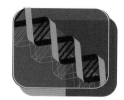

Preface

Progress in the field of genetics has moved at breakneck speed since the discovery of the structure of DNA in 1953. At that time, no human disease had been connected to our chromosomes or DNA. More than 50 years later, starting with the completion of the human genome project, the pace of discovery has only accelerated, moving quickly out of research into the clinic. Traditionally, diseases involving DNA were in the domain of genetics experts. But now, as the underpinnings of more and more conditions can be traced back to our genetic code, few fields of medicine can avoid this genomic revolution.

With revolutions and rapid change come challenges. Medical school curricula are still catching up with genomic medicine, and practicing physicians and other health professionals are left to educate themselves. Recalling our own training, we realized that students and residents don't read huge textbooks, but rather gravitate toward high yield, efficient, practical material. Unable to find such a guide for genomic and precision medicine, we endeavored to write it ourselves.

Providing a comprehensive overview of the practice of genomic medicine while keeping the material tight and concise was not simple and we struggled mightily to achieve the ideal scope in this handbook. There is a reason why existing texts are tomes: genomic knowledge is expansive. Therefore, this book is not intended for the genetics expert, nor does it provide a complete background in biology for a beginner. Rather, this text is intended for general health care practitioners and trainees (primary care, hospitalist, residents, nurses, and students in these and related disciplines) with two goals. First, the book offers detailed guidance on many applications of genomic medicine that have already penetrated nonspecialty medical care. Second, it provides background and practical knowledge on current and imminent technologies and concepts that will enhance a health care provider's confidence and efficiency when interacting with specialists, specialty tests, and informed patients. Throughout, we strive to highlight common pitfalls— technical and ethical—that might complicate the provision of quality genomic medical care. The emphasis is always on real-life patient interactions and decision support, though the reader must be cautioned that practices both vary and evolve and there are few simplicities.

Also for the sake of brevity, this text is necessarily selective about which aspects of genomic and precision medicine are considered. Many readers may find a specific topic inadequately addressed. For more in-depth information on a specific test or topic, we provide resources that can be consulted. We encourage feedback for future editions of the book. Our emphases for this inaugural edition are applications of genomic medicine that are common, commonly misunderstood, or involve recent technological innovations.

This book is divided by life stages, beginning before conception through adulthood. Several appendices detail subjects that span these categories, such as diagnostic technology, ethical issues, and the nuts-and-bolts of ordering tests. A pediatrician, for example, may be tempted to read only those chapters that pertain to children, but we would humbly suggest that he read the entire text. Important, common threads weave together the application of precision medicine at every life stage and inform each other.

A common theme in the coming chapters is a sea change in the practice of clinical genetics. In the past, eligibility for genetic testing was carefully calculated and such testing was only offered to clearly defined patients, usually because of a quantifiable risk (advanced maternal age, family history, etc.). This approach is eroding, replaced by a more consumer-driven model by which patients are considered to be entitled to whatever genomic information they desire, with the health care practitioner as a partner rather than a gatekeeper. Payers are also struggling to keep up with advancing technology and challenges with reimbursement abound.

The most extreme form of genetic accessibility is direct-to-consumer genomic testing, which is discussed further in Chapter 11. The wisdom and cost-effectiveness of this new approach will be the subject of debate for years to come. Even within the realm of physician-ordered testing, the emphasis has clearly shifted from deciding *if* a patient should get testing, to ensuring that testing is appropriately, consistently, and accurately applied and interpreted. The practice of Genomic and Precision medicine has not yet succeeded in achieving this objective, and this text is part of a larger effort to equip the nongeneticist practitioner with the background to apply genomic technology responsibly and for the betterment of patients.

If we could provide one piece of advice for anyone diving into the world of Genomic and Precision medicine for the first time: be skeptical but excited. Meet the skepticism with ambition to learn more, not avoidance or paralysis. Balance the excitement with a determination to provide the highest quality and evidence-based care possible, not an immediate acceptance of everything new. Within this equilibrium, the application of precision medicine can be of benefit to patients and providers alike.

Acknowledgements

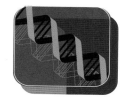

The authors would like to thank Mary Norton, Arun Wiita, Audrey Brumback, Jaekyu Shin, Susanne Haga, Mike McConnell, Joshua Knowles, Sherri Millis, Julie Mak, Erica Ramos, Wendy Rubinstein, Saivash Sarlati, and Kathryn Phillips for helpful review and comments.

Dr. McCarthy would like to thank the following mentors who inspired, supported and guided her throughout her scientific career: Therese Markow, Mary-Claire King and Geoff Ginsburg.

Dr. Mendelsohn would like to that those who have imparted their knowledge and enthusiasm for Genetics, including Anne Slavotinek, Renata Gallagher, Tony Wynshaw-Boris, Kate Rauen, Ophir Klein, Sy Packman, Joseph Shieh, and Bob Nussbaum.

FAMILY PLANNING AND PREGNANCY

PART

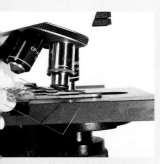
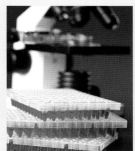
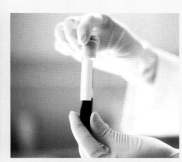
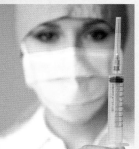
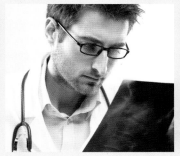
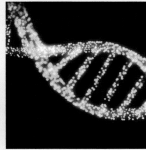

CHAPTER 1

Preconception Carrier Screening

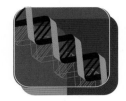

Even before a child is conceived, much (but certainly not all) of the information needed to determine a future child's risk of having a genetic disease is already present in the genomes of his or her parents. For dominant diseases, the parent may be affected and the concept of screening does not apply. For recessive diseases, parents can carry a pathogenic mutation in one of their genes and will typically be unaffected and unaware that they carry a mutation. But if a child inherits both pathogenic mutations from two carrier parents, they are at risk of the disease (refer to Appendix 3 for more information on inheritance). For this reason, much of the advancement in Genomic and Precision Medicine has occurred in the field of prenatal and preconception carrier testing of prospective parents. This chapter will deal with these advancements and their practical use by nongeneticist physicians and practitioners such as primary care providers, obstetricians, pediatricians, midwives, and fertility specialists.

Since the 1970s, tests have been available to detect carrier parents who might have a child affected by a rare recessive disease if the reproductive partner is also a carrier. Diseases such as Tay–Sachs have been almost eliminated in select populations due to aggressive carrier screening. However, screening for a small number of disorders in a narrow segment of the population is a far cry from screening all prospective parents for all medicine, but medicine is indeed heading in that direction.

TRADITIONAL CARRIER SCREENING

Carrier screening has traditionally been heavily influenced by pretest risk. Individuals with a family history of a genetic disorder would be offered carrier testing. Prospective parents belonging to a unique ethnic group with a higher rate of a particular disorder would be screened for that disorder only. Screening beyond this was simply not technically or financially feasible.

Now, the cost of sequencing many genes is essentially the same as sequencing one, and medicine has swung away from paternalism and seeks to involve the patient to whatever extent is possible and desired. These two forces have combined to fertilize (pun intended) a robust industry providing a variety of carrier screening products that detect an ever-increasing number of disorders, and that are marketed to any and all prospective parents regardless of family or ethnic background.

Nevertheless, obtaining a complete family history remains essential for any provider caring for a prospective parent. As will be discussed below, many of the newer one-size-fits-all commercial preconception screening tests are not necessarily suited for a family with a clear history of a specific disease. Diseases that run in the family, especially in children, may require testing and counseling by a specialist. It is the responsibility of the primary practitioner to distinguish families that lack defined risk factors for inherited diseases and can thus appropriately undergo generic screening from those families that require more in-depth consideration.

Perhaps the most important concept to recognize with carrier screening of any kind is that *the mother need not be pregnant to undergo testing*. Indeed, the reproductive options available to couples that carry the same disease are vastly more limited if the pregnancy has already commenced. For this reason, nonobstetrics practitioners should be on the front line of understanding and discussing carrier screening for any patients contemplating reproduction.

Table 1-1 shows the diseases currently recommended by the American College of Medical Genetics and Genomics (ACMG) for carrier screening of individuals regardless of family history (the American College of Obstetrics and Gynecology—ACOG—has a similar but shorter list; note that these recommendations may change with time).

> **Key Point**
>
> No advancement in preconception carrier screening will replace a quality family history. A practitioner must distinguish families that are candidates for one-size-fits-all carrier screening from those families that require further consideration, possibly with a specialist.

> **Key Point**
>
> Many more reproductive options are available to patients who are not already pregnant. Whenever possible, carrier screening should be offered *before pregnancy*. Practitioners such as obstetricians who see women after they are pregnant and routinely send carrier screening should seek out the primary care providers referring to them and educate about carrier screening.

EXPANDED CARRIER SCREENING (ECS)

Expanded carrier screening is the practice of testing men and women (often as partners) for more diseases than their family history or ethnicity specifically place them at elevated risk for carrying compared to the general population. Practically, ECS has taken the form of large panels that determine the carrier status for 100 or more conditions and are applied uniformly to any prospective parent. Universal guidelines for the use of ECS have not been established, but guidance is available[1].

Clinical utility of ECS

The evidence supporting the use of ECS as a universal screen for all prospective parents can best be described as incomplete. Studies have demonstrated[2] that ECS does in fact detect carriers who would not have been considered candidates for traditional risk-based screening, but this is not the same as saying that increased detection leads to better pregnancy outcomes. Studies examining common genetic diseases such as cystic fibrosis have suggested that merely screening for a disorder reduces its incidence in newborns, though it is not clear what proportion of this reduced incidence is due to reduced

Table 1-1. ACMG recommended diseases for carrier screening regardless of family history, by ancestry.

	Ashkenazi Jewish	Caucasian	African	Asian
Cystic fibrosis	✓	✓	✓	
Sickle cell anemia			✓	
Thalassemia		(Some)	✓	✓
Tay–Sachs	✓			
Canavan	✓			
Familial Dysautonomia	✓			
Fanconi anemia C	✓			
Niemann–Pick A	✓			
Mucolipidosis IV	✓			
Bloom syndrome	✓			
Gaucher disease	✓			
Spinal muscular atrophy	✓	✓	✓	✓

reproductive rates in carrier couples (i.e., couples choose not to have children), elective termination of affected pregnancies, or use of donor gametes or other reproductive technologies (see below)[3]. It is less clear how parents respond to more rare disorders they are unlikely to have encountered.

Another challenge with ECS panels is that the tested genes—and therefore diseases—vary widely in terms of clinical severity, penetrance, and the degree to which medical science understands their natural history and genotype–phenotype correlation (i.e., how well a particular mutation actually predicts disease severity and age of onset). As a consequence, for some diseases on these panels there will be considerable uncertainty as to if, when, and how badly a child might be affected if born to a given carrier couple. The lack of precise guidelines for including genes on ECS panels leaves ECS labs to their own devices to formulate their panels, which are in turn as imperfect as medical science's knowledge of countless rare diseases. For these and other reasons, expanded carrier screening for all prospective parents is not currently the standard of care.

Is ECS cost-effective?

On one hand, sequencing is expensive and screening whole populations for the rare couples that both carry the same disease requires a significant up-front cost before any clinical benefit can be realized. Some persons who discover that they are carriers may feel the need to see experts, undergo more advanced testing, and may experience anxiety leading to increased health care seeking behaviors, even if their partner does not carry the same disease. Those couples that both carry the same disease may pursue expensive reproductive technologies to have healthy children. As diseases or variants of less certain clinical relevance become included on ECS panels, parents and children might pursue lengthy testing odysseys without clear benefit.

On the other hand, the care of individuals born with rare inherited disorders can be enormously expensive, not to mention the loss of quality of life—for all parties—associated with many serious illnesses. Medical practices that improve health outcomes can be justified even if costs increase simply because good health is worth paying for. More study is needed to place ECS in the context of other medical interventions in terms of cost-effectiveness, and such studies are complicated by the fact that the cost of sequencing and the size and diagnostic yield of ECS panels are rapidly moving targets.

The general expectation is that ECS can and will be either cost-effective or worth the cost, but realizing this goal will require: (1) the continuing decline in the cost of sequencing, (2) thoughtful and responsible inclusion and exclusion of diseases (and reported variants) in ECS panels, (3) excellent patient counseling and education before and after testing, and (4) careful clinical follow up of the downstream decisions and outcomes of parents who undergo ECS and their children.

Guidance for ECS

The ACMG, ACOG, and several other important organizations involved in reproductive genetics issued a joint statement providing some guidance regarding ECS panels. These are useful to review as they highlight some of the major limitations and risks associated with ECS panels[1,4]. We recommend reviewing these references. Some major points are summarized here:

1. Diseases should be sufficiently clinically significant that parents would want to know about them. Testing for mild diseases or those that do not affect every child, for example, may create more anxiety, cost, or even unnecessary pregnancy termination than any potential benefit. Most current panels contain at least a few genes whose associated disease could be classified as mild. For example, alpha-1-antitrypsin deficiency is included on many ECS panels, but the severity and age-of-onset for disease symptoms associated with this condition is highly variable and often after childhood.

2. Testing for adult-onset diseases should be done with caution, as results may reveal unexpected and unwanted clinically significant disease risk for the parent. Example: *BRCA1* testing. Identifying such a mutation on carrier screening would have immediate health implications for the mother, which might be unexpected and unwelcomed if she had not been properly counseled before testing and thought she was only testing for disease

that might affect a future child. Infrequently, parents are found by ECS to be affected by a recessive or X-linked disorder that was unrecognized.

3. As much as possible should be known about the gene(s), mutations, and mutation frequencies for a disease in a patient's population so that accurate counseling about risk and residual risk can be provided. **Residual risk** is an acknowledgment of the inability of any genetic test to identify 100% of disease-causing mutations, and thus reflects the possibility that a parent who screened negative for a disorder is actually a carrier (i.e., a false-negative screen). The residual risk calculation depends on the patient's ethnic group (likelihood of being a carrier before any testing) and the probability the test missed a mutation, which will vary by the gene and the methodology used for the screening panel. Residual risk should be communicated in any ECS report. Calculation of residual risk is hindered if the reproductive partner is not known.

4. In the unique case of Tay–Sachs, non-Ashkenazi partners of known carriers should have enzyme testing, not sequencing.

5. More work is needed to define the costs and benefits of ECS to identify the ideal means to educate patients and providers, and to formalize the types of reproductive decisions and outcomes that might be influenced by ECS.

Questions to ask about a carrier screening test

Does this test sequence entire genes, or only genotype known mutations?

*   Refer to Appendix 2 for a complete discussion of the difference between sequencing and genotyping.
*   Sequencing the entire gene is more comprehensive, but also more likely to find variants of uncertain significance (VUS), and thus can lead to the misinterpretation that the parent carries a disease (false-positive). Companies that offer testing vary in how they report these VUS, but generally (and ideally) do not report these.
*   Sequencing only previously recognized mutations might lead to false-negatives because less common mutations are not detected, particularly in ethnicities that have a different spectrum of mutations than those covered by the test. On the other hand, for some well-studied ethnic groups (e.g., Ashkenazi Jews), nearly all cases of a few specific diseases are attributable to a small number of known mutations and targeted mutation testing is essentially as sensitive as full-gene sequencing.

What diseases does the test cover, and how many?

*   More isn't necessarily better. Some diseases are mild or can start only later in life. Tests that partially sequence a greater number of genes may miss more disease-causing mutations than tests that comprehensively

sequence fewer genes, but this is difficult to compare quantitatively. The bottom line is that little evidence exists to scientifically compare currently available commercial carrier screening panels.

- The composition of carrier screening panels changes so rapidly it is not possible to comment on individual companies' tests in detail in this text.
- If the parents are interested in a specific disease or diseases, be sure these are included on a panel before ordering.

Practice Point: Clinical Counseling

Sample counseling before ECS:

"From our conversation today, it sounds like you are thinking about starting a family and want to know more about genetic tests that can help you learn your risk for having a child affected by a genetic disease. There are tests available for just that purpose, but there is important information you need to know about before undergoing testing.

The purpose of carrier screening is to determine if you carry any changes in your DNA that might cause a disease in your child. These diseases usually don't make you sick, and your reproductive partner would have to carry the same disease in order for your future child to be affected. This information can be very empowering if it is desired, because there are options available to couples who both carry the same disease to help them have healthy children. But carrier screening isn't perfect, so let's make sure you understand the limitations and what results you might get.

First, no genetic test can identify 100% of changes in our DNA that might cause a disease in a child, and no available test today looks at every gene in the genome. So, you must understand that carrier screening can only be used to *reduce* the risk of having a child with *some* diseases.

Second, many genetic diseases such as Trisomy 21 (Down syndrome) are caused by random errors in the particular egg or sperm that formed the baby, and cannot be detected by ECS.

Third, a small number of the diseases on these panels can cause health problems even in carriers, and so you might find unexpected information about your own health. Think about if you would want to know this type of information.

Fourth, almost every human being carries at least one genetic disease, so there's a good chance your test will come back 'positive' for a disease. Unless your partner carries the same disease there is little risk to your children, so you should not be worried if you do carry a disease. If you want to pursue screening, we can test just you today, and only test your partner if you carry something. This might be less expensive, but think about how you will feel waiting for results to come back on your partner if you are found to carry a disease, which is likely. If you think this would be nerve-wracking, we can consider testing both of you simultaneously.

If you do carry a disease, others in your family may carry the same disease, so you should think about whether and how you would share this information with them. I can help you with that if you wish.

The last thing I want to ask you is if there are any diseases that run in your family, particularly in children. If there is a genetic disease in your family, I may need to talk to a specialist to be sure that the ECS test I order is right for that disease.

Do you have any questions?"

What support is offered for the test and results?

- For those practitioners ordering the test who do not feel comfortable discussing the diseases on the panel should results return positive, the testing lab (or the practitioner's own colleagues/hospital) could provide needed support.

Is reanalysis available?

- The classification of variants as disease-causing or not changes over time as more information is accumulated. Ask if the testing lab offers to reissue its report with up-to-date information and at what cost.

Are diseases relevant to my patient on this panel?

- If the family is from an ethnicity that has a higher frequency of a particular set of disorders, determine if the panel covers these diseases. If it is a targeted mutation panel, determine if the common mutation(s) present in that population are covered.

ECS: When to proceed with caution

Sometimes providing personalized medicine means *not* sending advanced genomic tests. Such circumstances might include:

- If the family does not wish to know their carrier status for genetic diseases. Note that wishing to know carrier status is not equivalent to being willing to terminate an affected pregnancy.
- If the family has a history of a disease and the practitioner is not certain that this disease is adequately covered by an expanded carrier screening panel.
- If the family has clearly articulated that they only wish to determine if they carry a specific disease or set of diseases: for example, an Ashkenazi-Jewish couple who only wants to know their risk of diseases clearly enriched in this population. More limited genetic testing would be appropriate in this situation.

What to expect from ECS results

As more genes are being added to ECS panels, and as they are sequenced more completely, the odds are increasing that an ECS panel will show that the patient does carry at least one disorder. This is not surprising, as genomic studies suggest that most humans carry at least one, and often multiple, recessive Mendelian diseases[2]. There are several ways to mitigate any negative psychological consequences of having a positive screen:

- Counsel the patient before testing that there is a reasonable chance (about 35% for Counsyl's panel, though the exact percentage varies by the panel, the patient's ethnicity, and will change as more genes are added) that he or she will carry one or more diseases, and that this is normal and common. Remind the patient that carrying a recessive disease primarily will be of concern if their reproductive partner carries the same disease, which is rare.

- For cost and efficiency reasons, unless a pregnancy is already quite advanced, a common approach is to test a couple sequentially, only testing the other partner if the first partner (usually the mother) is found to carry a disease. Because an individual will be found to carry a disease about one-third of the time with current panels, there may be a period of anxiety while the other partner's test is pending. This eventuality must be discussed and the costs of simultaneous testing (which will vary by insurance) weighed against the couple's feelings about waiting for a second test to return. This is particularly true if a pregnancy has already begun. As will be much repeated, carrier screening is ideally conducted before a pregnancy begins.

- Encourage the parents to think about if and how they would talk to their family members should they find out that they carry a disease. Some individuals prefer to keep all genetic information private. Others, perhaps with reproductive age siblings, would wish to share their test results with their families to help them make reproductive decisions.

- Become familiar with the diseases on the panel, especially the more common ones. This will allow the parents' questions to be answered efficiently when results return.

- Identify a specialist who can be available to counsel patients and provide detailed information about diseases in the event that the parents' needs exceed the knowledge and experience of the nongeneticist practitioner.

> **Key Point**
>
> One common question asked when only one parent is found to carry a recessive genetic condition is "after our baby is born, can he get tested to see if he is also a carrier like I am." The answer to this question is usually, "*yes, but because his carrier status will not affect his health as a child, he can choose to find out after he turns 18 and decides he wants to know this information.*" See Appendix 9 for a more complete discussion of the ethics of genetic testing in minors.

In the uncommon circumstance that both members of a couple carry the same genetic disease (or a woman carries an X-linked disorder), there are a variety of reproductive options. None is perfect, and the preference of families will vary greatly depending on cost, attitudes toward abortion, and the value they place on having their own biological children.

Options for families:

- Not having biological children/adopting.
- Using donor gametes (sperm or egg). Some services will offer testing of the donor for the genetic condition of interest. This option necessitates that one parent will not be a biological parent.
- "Taking their chances." Conceived naturally, each fetus would have a 75% chance of being unaffected (for most conditions), which may be an

acceptable risk to some families. If desired, prenatal testing is possible to determine if the fetus is affected.

- Conceiving naturally, and testing the fetus with the intent to terminate if the fetus is affected. See Chapter 2 for approaches to reaching a prenatal diagnosis.

- Preimplantation genetic diagnosis (PGD). This method involves in vitro fertilization with gametes from both carrier parents, then before implanting embryos, a single cell is tested from several embryos to identify unaffected embryos, which are then implanted. The benefit of this approach is that it does not involve terminating an implanted pregnancy (though families that consider life to begin at conception may consider it equivalent), while allowing the couples to have children biologically related to both parents with a very low risk of being affected by the disorder. The primary downside is cost; a single round of PGD can cost several tens of thousands of dollars. PGD is sometimes covered by insurance, but the IVF is often not. Also, the woman is subjected to hormonal treatments necessary for IVF that carry small medical risks.

> **Key Point**
>
> ECS should not be used to evaluate an abnormal fetus, or to diagnose a genetic condition in a parent. ECS is intended as a screen, not a diagnostic test.

FUTURE OF CARRIER SCREENING AND PRECONCEPTION GENETICS

For the near future, progress in the application of ECS primarily will involve larger and larger gene panels that sequence more of each gene. Private insurers largely are covering carrier screening and it is likely that public insurance (Medicaid in the United States) eventually will follow suit. Unless a seismic shift in the funding of health care in the United States occurs, it is probable that any remaining eligibility requirements for carrier screening will evaporate, and large gene panels could eventually be applied universally to all prospective parents.

Several challenges will be created by the much wider application of ECS. How do we maximize the number of parents who get screened *before* pregnancy? How do we optimally educate parents and providers to be sure everyone receives the desired test and excellent pre and posttest counseling? Can we make ECS available despite insurance limitations? Will there be evidence that ECS reduces recessive disease burden or infant mortality? What if ECS increases health care costs? Will gene panels reflect our best understanding of the severity and treatability of each condition[5]?

Other challenges come after a couple finds that they carry the same disease. Insurance coverage is limited for PGD or IVF. As screening increases, demand for these services also will increase. How insurers will handle the demand for expensive reproductive services (raising rates, enforcing strict eligibility criteria) remains to be seen. Also, as more diseases are added to panels, the selection of diseases to include may encroach on gray areas of diseases that are more mild, have a later onset, or have lower penetrance, leading to debates as to which disorders are fair grounds to base reproductive decisions, and who gets to make these decisions.

As the number of genes tested by ECS panels increases, there will be a blurring of purpose as some diseases that might affect the carrier parent, such as dominant or late-onset diseases, are included. Indeed, carrier screening is likely to merge with other genetic screening intended to benefit the patient/parent directly. This would consist of a single genetic test that provides useful information about heart disease, diet, and medications to avoid, and also covers recessive disorders for reproductive purposes. At what age this test would be offered, who would initiate it (the patient or physician), and how results and counseling will be delivered to large numbers of patients are all challenges for the future.

Table 1-2 provides a nonexhaustive list of the current commercially available ECS panels in no particular order (no endorsement is made of any test). Note that tests change rapidly, insurance coverage varies, and we encourage the reader to compare several of these panels based on the comments above.

Table 1-2. Nonexhaustive list of currently available commercial ECS panels.

Company	Test	Link
Sequenom	HerediT® UNIVERSAL	https://laboratories.sequenom.com/providers/heredit-universal/
Counsyl	Family Prep Screen	https://www.counsyl.com/services/family-prep-screen/
Recombine	CarrierMap	https://recombine.com/carriermap
Natera	Horizon™ Carrier Screen	http://www.natera.com/reproductive-genetic-testing
Pathway Genomics	DNA Insight®	https://www.pathway.com/carrier-status-dna-insight/
LabCorp (Integrated Genetics)	Inheritest℠	http://www.integratedgenetics.com/
Emory Genetics Laboratory	Pan-Ethnic Carrier Screen	http://geneticslab.emory.edu/about/news-and-events/news/2014/06/pan-ethnic-carrier-screen/index.html
Baylor Miraca Genetics Laboratories	GeneAware	https://geneaware.clinical.bcm.edu/GeneAware/default.aspx

Practice Point: Clinical Scenario

A couple would like to start a family and comes to the office for the first time to establish care with an obstetrician. The future mother and father are not related to each other to their knowledge. The father reveals that his full brother died in childhood of Zellweger syndrome, a rare recessive Mendelian disorder. They would like to know what options are available to be sure a future child is not affected by Zellweger.

Consider the following:

1. Are they interested primarily in learning about Zellweger, or about other inherited diseases?
2. Even if they are interested in learning about other disorders as well, do any ECS panels include any or all known Zellweger genes? Does the father know which Zellweger gene was affected in his brother? (Mutations in multiple genes can cause Zellweger syndrome.)
3. Does the father know the mutation(s) that caused Zellweger in his family? If so it would be straightforward to determine if he is a carrier (2/3 chance).
4. If the gene/mutations are not known, what would be a reasonable approach, and who would carry out this evaluation? Samples from the deceased brother (if available), the father, the father's parents, or the mother could all be used to inform the risk of a future pregnancy being affected.

REFERENCES

1. Edwards JG, Feldman G, Goldberg J, et al. Expanded carrier screening in reproductive medicine-points to consider: a joint statement of the American College of Medical Genetics and Genomics, American College of Obstetricians and Gynecologists, National Society of Genetic Counselors, Perinatal Quality Foundation, and Society for Maternal-Fetal Medicine. *Obstet Gynecol.* 2015;125(3):653-662. doi:10.1097/AOG.0000000000000666.
2. Lazarin GA, Haque IS, Nazareth S, et al. An empirical estimate of carrier frequencies for 400+ causal Mendelian variants: results from an ethnically diverse clinical sample of 23,453 individuals. *Genet Med.* 2013;15(3):178-186. doi:10.1038/gim.2012.114.
3. Castellani C, Picci L, Tamanini A, Girardi P, Rizzotti P, Assael BM. Association between carrier screening and incidence of cystic fibrosis. *JAMA.* 2009;302(23):2573-2579. doi:10.1001/jama.2009.1758.
4. Grody WW, Thompson BH, Gregg AR, et al. ACMG position statement on prenatal/preconception expanded carrier screening. *Genet Med.* 2013;15(6):482-483. doi:10.1038/gim.2013.47.
5. Grimes DA, Schulz KF. Uses and abuses of screening tests. *Lancet.* 2002;359(9309):881-884. doi:10.1016/S0140-6736(02)07948-5.

CHAPTER 2

Pregnancy

For decades, the only application of genetic screening that most individuals would ever encounter was testing for aneuploidies in pregnant women, particularly those over age 35. The risk of a fetus being affected by Trisomy 21 (discussed as a clinical entity in Chapter 3) increases gradually as a woman ages, and 35 was somewhat arbitrarily selected as the age at which the risk of Trisomy 21 was sufficiently high to justify testing by amniocentesis or chorionic villus sampling (CVS), each of which carries with it a very small risk of miscarriage or other fetal complications. However, the majority of children with Trisomy 21 are born to women younger than 35, simply because younger women have disproportionately more children than their reduced risk for Trisomy 21.

INTEGRATED SCREENING

Less invasive testing has become common practice for women of any age that relies on ultrasound imaging of the fetus (looking for specific characteristics of Trisomy 21 and nuchal translucency, which can be increased in many conditions), and by measuring some combination of alpha-fetoprotein (AFP), estriol, PAPP-A, inhibin, and/or beta-human chorionic gonadotropin (beta-hCG) in the mother's blood. For sequential integrated screening, a first blood draw occurs between 10 and 14 weeks of gestation, the second blood draw between 15 and 20 weeks, with a measurement of nuchal translucency between approximately 11 and 14 weeks. Variations include a single blood draw between 15 and 20 weeks (quad screening), or serum integrated screening (both blood samples without measuring nuchal translucency). Based on the mother's age, these values are used to calculate a modified risk of Trisomy 21, neural tube defects, and a small number of additional conditions in the fetus, and to determine if amniocentesis or further ultrasound imaging might be indicated to rule in or out a diagnosis.

A major advantage of integrated screening is that it relies on physical and serum-based markers that can be disturbed by a range of fetal abnormalities. Mosaic aneuploidies, subchromosomal insertions and deletions, translocations, neural tube defects, and Smith–Lemli–Opitz syndrome are examples of conditions that are still only detectable by integrated screening with follow-up invasive diagnostic testing. Integrated screening is also relatively inexpensive compared to sequencing-based technologies.

These tests should be familiar to any obstetric practitioner and have been available for many years. This type of integrated screening will not be discussed in detail in this text. Also familiar to any who regularly employ this type of screening is the limited specificity of these tests. Sensing a commercial opportunity in prenatal screening, research was directed at improving the sensitivity and specificity of prenatal testing for aneuploidies.

NONINVASIVE PRENATAL SCREENING (NIPS, AKA CELL-FREE DNA SCREENING)

Several high-profile publications have recently highlighted the utility of noninvasive prenatal screening (NIPS) based on cell-free DNA (cfDNA) as a means to detect trisomies[1,2]. After approximately seven weeks of gestation, as much as 10% of the free-floating DNA in a pregnant woman's blood is from the placenta of her fetus. By sequencing regions of each chromosome many times from this cfDNA, a quantitative measurement of the abundance of each chromosome is obtained and allows one to determine statistically how much of each chromosome is present in the cfDNA fraction in the mother's blood. A subtle excess of one chromosome could be an indication of a trisomy in the placenta, and therefore the fetus.

Clinical utility

For the detection of Trisomy 21, NIPS is a substantially more specific test when compared to traditional integrated screening based on nuchal translucency and/or protein analysis. In one recent study of low-risk pregnancies, the positive predictive value of NIPS for Trisomy 21 was 80.9% compared to 3.4% for standard screening and NIPS had a false-positive rate of 0.06% compared to 5.4% for standard screening. Better, however, is still not perfect. Compared to amniocentesis or CVS (the gold standards), NIPS still produces some false-positive and negative results, and current guidelines clearly state that a woman with a positive NIPS should be offered CVS or amniocentesis before making any decisions regarding pregnancy termination. Causes of false-positive NIPS results include subchromosomal copy number variants in the mother or fetus (which can be pathogenic or benign)[3], aneuploidy restricted to the placenta, and even undetected maternal cancer.

NIPS caveats and limitations

NIPS has some other limitations compared to traditional integrated screening. First, a small but important percentage of pregnancies (about 3%) yield uninterpretable results from NIPS[4]. In this study, the frequency of genetic abnormalities was higher in the uninterpretable group, but most of the fetuses were normal. A common cause of uninterpretable results was a low fraction of fetal DNA. Maternal obesity has also been associated with an increased risk of NIPS failure. How these cases are handled represents a major unresolved component of the performance of NIPS.

If uninterpretable results are viewed as negatives, then the true sensitivity of the NIPS test is lower than reported above. If they are viewed as positives (i.e., more testing is performed on the pregnancy), then the positive predictive value of NIPS alone would decrease. Until these scenarios are better understood and handled by the technology, a fraction of women undergoing NIPS will receive uncertain and possibly anxiety-provoking results. Many recommend repeating NIPS or offering invasive testing to clarify these uninterpretable or uninformative results.

NIPS also is being used increasingly to detect subchromosomal deletions, such as DiGeorge syndrome (22q11.2 deletion). Detection of such deletions would be clinically important because, like Trisomy 21, they often are de novo events that cannot usually be detected by carrier screening in the parents, yet can be phenotypically as severe as a trisomy. The accurate detection of such deletions should theoretically be technically feasible, but currently this technology is quite new and caution is warranted. Perhaps the major challenge is that microdeletion syndromes (with the possible exception of 22q11.2) are so much rarer than trisomies. Recall from Appendix 7 that the same test will have different positive predictive values depending on the frequency of the disorder being screened. Therefore, it would be very difficult to achieve an acceptable positive predictive value (see Appendix 7) for microdeletions with current technology. In fact, organizations such as the American College of Obstetrics and Gynecology (ACOG) recommend against using NIPS to screen for microdeletions. Inaccurate screens have been reported in the literature, and studies as to the sensitivity and specificity of microdeletion screening (which are only recently emerging for trisomies) are almost entirely lacking.

Another area of controversy with NIPS is screening for sex chromosome abnormalities. Physical and cognitive phenotypes of individuals with 47,XXX or 47,XYY karyotypes can be mild and overlap with normal, raising the dilemma of screening (and possibly terminating) these pregnancies.

SUMMARY

Noninvasive screening of pregnancies undoubtedly will continue to advance, and current practices vary widely while quality evidence comparing prenatal screening paradigms is only recently becoming available. ACOG has released guidelines on the use of NIPS[5]. Rather than adhere to a single set of guidelines, the following are suggestions for the use of NIPS given the reality of modern practice.

- Patients should receive counseling before testing is sent, covering the purpose of the NIPS screen, limitations, the possible results (including "uninformative" or "uninterpretable") with a discussion of what next steps might be necessary depending on results. NIPS only screens for a small number of potential genetic conditions in a fetus.

- Increasingly, NIPS is being added to integrated screening for all pregnant women, but doing so probably oversimplifies its costs and benefits. Ordering both tests, particularly in younger women, is unlikely to be cost-effective[6], given the lower risk for trisomies and therefore low pretest probability, and has not been shown to improve pregnancy outcomes. In older mothers (about 40 years) where the risk of trisomies becomes greater than other abnormalities not detected by NIPS, testing routinely with NIPS is more justifiable. This is a rapidly evolving topic worth following closely.

- NIPS can be used to follow up a positive integrated screen for Trisomy 21, and doing so may reduce the need for invasive procedures when NIPS is negative. The use of NIPS versus going directly to invasive testing to follow up positive integrated screens must be individualized.

- Some woman may prefer (or maternal age and other factors may indicate) a more comprehensive genetic evaluation that is currently possible only with invasive diagnostic testing, making NIPS superfluous.

- Abnormal results from NIPS should not be considered diagnostic on their own. No management decision should be based on NIPS alone.

- NIPS should not be used to evaluate abnormalities detected on ultrasound. Diagnostic testing should be offered (CVS/amniocentesis with array, karyotype, or other tests).

- NIPS should be used with great caution to detect microdeletions until better data are available on the sensitivity and specificity of this use.

- NIPS should be used with caution with multiple gestations.

- Women may reasonably decline all aneuploidy screening.

- No genetic test guarantees a healthy pregnancy and baby.

Practice Point: Clinical Counseling

Sample counseling before offering NIPS:

"Congratulations on your pregnancy! As you may have already experienced, being pregnant can come with the desire to know if you are carrying a healthy baby, and many women opt for prenatal screening tests to identify some common genetic conditions that can affect your baby's health. Some women choose not to undergo screening at all. You should think about whether you want this kind of information, and what decisions you might make based on this information.

Your risk of a trisomy such as Trisomy 21 is approximately ____ based on your age, but further testing would be necessary to determine if the risk to this particular pregnancy is higher or lower than that. This choice is yours to make if you want to know more about your baby's health.

You may have heard of a new test called noninvasive prenatal testing or screening (NIPT or NIPS). This is a test where we take your blood (not your baby's) and run a complex DNA test that looks for extra chromosomes in the baby. When it comes to detecting extra chromosomes, this test is better than older technologies in that it doesn't as often suggest a problem when there isn't one, but it has some important limitations. It costs more, and depending on your insurance, may be expensive for you. It doesn't test for as many problems in a fetus as does more traditional testing. Sometimes it doesn't give a result at all and we may have to consider further testing. Rarely, it can reveal something quite unexpected, such as a difference in your chromosomes or even an undetected cancer. Most importantly, NIPS isn't perfect and if it shows evidence of a chromosomal abnormality, we may need to do an invasive test like amniocentesis to know with confidence if the NIPS test was correct."

Table 2-1. Nonexhaustive list of diagnostic labs offering NIPS.

Laboratory	Test	Link
Ariosa Diagnostics	Harmony™ Prenatal Test	http://www.ariosadx.com/
Sequenom Laboratories	MATERNIT21®	https://laboratories.sequenom.com/providers/maternit21-plus/
Counsyl	Informed Pregnancy Screen	https://www.counsyl.com/services/informed-pregnancy-screen/
Natera	Panorama®	www.panoramatest.com/
Illumina (formerly Verinata)	verifi Prenatal Test	http://www.illumina.com/clinical/reproductive-genetic-health/nipt.html
Progenity	verfi®	http://progenity.com/non-invasive-prenatal-testing

Table 2-1 shows a nonexhaustive list of diagnostic labs offering NIPS. The labs are in no particular order and no endorsement is made of any laboratory.

CVS AND AMNIOCENTESIS

Chorionic villus sampling and amniocentesis are established invasive approaches to obtain fetal/placental tissue for genetic diagnosis. They remain the gold standards for confirming most diagnoses suggested by less invasive screening modalities. Nearly all genetic tests that can be performed ex utero also can be performed on tissues from derived CVS or amniocentesis (see Appendix 2 for a more in-depth discussion of such tests). It is worth noting the following differences regarding the use of genetic testing at the prenatal stage compared to postnatal testing:

- Many genome-wide tests are less available or modified for prenatal use. For example, whole exome sequencing rarely is used prenatally. Microarray testing is performed routinely, but cutoffs for reporting copy number variants usually are more stringent (i.e., smaller variants are less likely to be reported). These practices stem from a greater hesitancy to report uncertain variants that may not be able to be adequately evaluated in utero and thus force parents and obstetricians to make difficult choices about pregnancy management with incomplete data.

- Tests with a long turnaround time are rarely applied to prenatal samples because results may not return in time to make management decisions about a pregnancy, and labs do not want the pressure of needing to report results on a tight timetable.

- Testing for known family mutations (usually 1 or 2) is highly preferred for prenatal samples because results can be obtained quickly and are readily interpretable.
- Karyotypes are among the most commonly performed tests on CVS or amniocentesis tissue. Because CVS samples the placenta and not the fetus, it is not uncommon for a trisomy to be detected that is confined to the placenta. Amniocentesis, which samples mostly fetal cells, can be performed a few weeks later to distinguish between a true trisomy and a confined placental trisomy. A phenotypically normal child with a normal karyotype on amniocentesis does not need additional postnatal testing because a trisomy was detected in the placenta. In some cases, a confined placental trisomy can increase the risk of intrauterine growth restriction and/or preeclampsia.

PREIMPLANTATION GENETIC DIAGNOSIS

Preimplantation genetic diagnosis (PGD) was discussed in Chapter 1 as an option for parents to select embryos that do not harbor a genetic change that might cause disease. A full consideration of this technique is beyond the scope of this text, but a few key points are worth noting.

First and foremost, PGD requires that the genetic condition in question be understood at the molecular level, that is, the exact mutation or chromosomal translocation must be known. For families seeking to use this technology because of a previously affected child, this can be an important justification for aggressive diagnostic testing in the affected child.

In some PGD procedures, intracytoplasmic sperm injection (ICSI) of a harvested oocyte is performed to eliminate the possibility that a nonfertilizing sperm will be collected and genetically analyzed. Some techniques test the polar body of the egg, but this only addresses the maternal genetic and chromosomal contribution. In other approaches, the growing embryo is biopsied after a few days of development. This procedure can detect contributions from both parents, but may be confounded by chromosomal mosaicism that is common at these early embryonic stages. Perhaps the greatest current drawback of PGD is its cost, often tens-of-thousands of dollars per cycle without a guarantee that any cycle will result in a successful pregnancy. Despite these challenges, PGD offers a means to avoid genetic disease that does not require terminating an implanted pregnancy, a moral distinction that will be important to some parents.

Preimplantation genetic screening (PGS) is a related technique that does not seek to diagnose a single disorder but rather to screen for many disorders[7]. At this time, PGS is limited to screening for aneuploidies, often with the hope of improving pregnancy rates given that aneuploidies are a major cause of early miscarriage. Data still are emerging as to the success, cost-effectiveness, and risk/benefit calculations of different types of PGS.

Theoretically PGS could be used to screen for any number of genetic conditions, and the ethical employment of this technology is a topic of ongoing consideration. In the United States, PGD is not regulated by the government, and questionable practices such as sex selection do occur. Laws vary in other countries. If prices drop and PGD becomes more widely used, increased scrutiny may be inevitable.

PRENATAL SCREENING: WHEN TO SCREEN, TO SCREEN AT ALL?

Many pregnant women are screened for trisomies without a detailed discussion of their values and goals regarding the pregnancy. At least one study suggests that women given educational materials about the process of aneuploidy screening are more likely to opt out of invasive screening or screening altogether[8]. Before even broaching the complex topics of the different screening modalities available, one would be wise to start at a more basic level, probing the woman's or couple's desire for knowledge about the health of the pregnancy.

Having discussed both established and newer technologies for detecting fetal trisomies, it is appropriate to pause to put such screening into a larger context. Why is screening for trisomies so central to prenatal care?

The answer is primarily historical rather than scientific. For years, trisomies were the only type of genetic disorder that could be clearly detected by available tests and that were of relevance to all women regardless of family history. As clinical entities, none of the viable trisomies (trisomy X, Y, 13, 18, 21) are particularly unique. They span the full clinical spectrum from essentially normal to universally lethal, as would any random selection of single gene disorders. Trisomies, particularly Trisomy 21, are indeed more common than most single gene disorders, and they do affect different ethnicities equivalently. Beyond this, though, trisomies are not special types of genetic disease, and soon emerging technologies will permit any type of genetic condition to be screened for in any pregnancy (and ideally before a pregnancy, when possible). Broader screening may be welcomed, but a word of caution: high rates of false-positive and negative results remain a major shortcoming of prenatal screening, and if multiplied across countless more diseases they could generate an untenable screening regime and follow up testing. Medicine must be careful to apply these new technologies with wisdom and care.

FUTURE OF PRENATAL SCREENING

NIPS is primarily being used to detect aneuploidies only. However, sequencing can also be used to detect the presence of a number of other genetic disorders caused by mutations or copy number variations smaller than a whole chromosome. NIPS eventually will begin to overlap with ECS as a prenatal screen for any genetic disease. Because the fetus's genome has been established, de novo mutations inaccessible to ECS will be detectable only by NIPS or other tests of the fetus. As discussed, aneuploidies are not clinically more severe than many other single gene disorders, and by screening for more diverse conditions parents and providers will be able to learn much more about the genetic health of a fetus than was ever possible previously.

However, should NIPS begin to test for non-de novo genetic diseases (i.e., dominant or recessive inherited), we will run the risk of offering screening too late. Inherited diseases are detectable in the parents' genomes before the fetus is conceived, and because there are many more reproductive options available prior to conception, every effort should be made to educate prospective parents that carrier screening ideally should be performed before a pregnancy starts. Technically, the same concept of the optimal time for testing can be applied to newborn screening, discussed further in Chapter 3. Advancements in preconception and prenatal screening will be fascinating to observe.

Practice Point: Clinical Scenario 1

A 25-year-old woman who is 10 weeks pregnant would like to undergo "the new Down syndrome test" she has read about. There has been no other testing or imaging in the pregnancy.

Consider the following:

1. Does her insurance cover cfDNA (NIPS) testing? Would her out-of-pocket cost be acceptable to her?
2. Would she also be an appropriate candidate for integrated serum screening, given that this detects some disorders not covered by NIPS?
3. What are her feelings about the pregnancy and what would she do with an abnormal (uninterpretable or positive) result from NIPS?
4. Are there other indications from the pregnancy or family history that suggest that other testing might be appropriate?

Practice Point: Clinical Scenario 2

A 39-year-old woman has had NIPS (cfDNA screening) that returned with uninterpretable results. What comes next?

Consider the following:

1. How far along is the pregnancy, and is there urgency to identify or rule out a chromosomal disorder?
2. The NIPS could be repeated, or invasive testing could be performed. What case can be made for each approach in this individual?

REFERENCES

1. Norton ME, Wapner RJ. Cell-free DNA analysis for noninvasive examination of trisomy. *N Engl J Med*. 2015;373(26):2582. doi:10.1056/NEJMc1509344
2. Bianchi DW, Parker RL, Wentworth J, et al. DNA sequencing versus standard prenatal aneuploidy screening. *N Engl J Med*. 2014;370(9):799-808. doi:10.1056/NEJMoa1311037
3. Snyder MW, Simmons LE, Kitzman JO, et al. Copy-number variation and false positive prenatal aneuploidy screening results. *N Engl J Med*. 2015;372(17):1639-1645. doi:10.1056/NEJMoa1408408
4. Gil MM, Quezada MS, Revello R, Akolekar R, Nicolaides KH. Analysis of cell-free DNA in maternal blood in screening for fetal aneuploidies: updated meta-analysis. *Ultrasound Obstet Gynecol*. 2015;45(3):249-266. doi:10.1002/uog.14791
5. Committee Opinion No. 640: cell-free DNA screening for fetal aneuploidy. *Obstet Gynecol*. 2015;126(3):e31-e37. doi:10.1097/AOG.0000000000001051
6. Kaimal AJ, Norton ME, Kuppermann M. Prenatal testing in the genomic age: clinical outcomes, quality of life, and costs. *Obstet Gynecol*. 2015;126 (4):737-746. doi:10.1097/AOG.0000000000001029
7. Brezina PR, Ke RW, Kutteh WH. Preimplantation genetic screening: a practical guide. *Clin Med Insights Reprod Health*. 2013;7:37-42. doi:10.4137/CMRH.S10852
8. Kuppermann M, Pena S, Bishop JT, et al. Effect of enhanced information, values clarification, and removal of financial barriers on use of prenatal genetic testing: a randomized clinical trial. *JAMA*. 2014;312(12):1210-1217. doi:10.1001/jama.2014.11479

CHILDHOOD

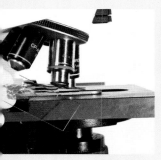
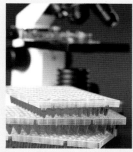
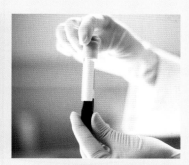
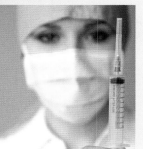
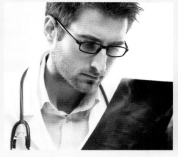
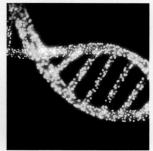

CHAPTER 3

The Newborn

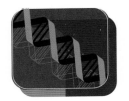

The diagnosis and management of Mendelian (i.e., single gene) dysmorphic or metabolic syndromes in newborns and children constitutes a major branch of the classical practice of Medical Genetics. Though the care and study of rare diseases in children also is being revolutionized by advances in genetic technologies, Mendelian genetics has long been a mature clinical field. Therefore, even a cursory overview of the accumulated knowledge of the diagnosis and care of Mendelian disorders in children would enormously exceed the scope of this book. Rather, in keeping with its goals, the aim of this and following chapters will be to (1) empower nongeneticist practitioners with a rational approach to the child with a suspected genetic disorder, (2) demystify the typical evaluation of a suspected disorder by a specialist, and (3) describe critical areas of recent or anticipated advancement where the nongeneticist will likely play an increasingly important role in applying genomic technologies to the care of children.

The essential first step whenever a genetic disorder is suspected is to conduct a detailed family history. A proper family history includes at least three generations: the child and all siblings, parents and all their siblings, uncles/aunts and first cousins, and the grandparents. In addition to determining the health of each relative and the cause of any deaths, it is important to ask about miscarriages/stillbirths, developmental delay, seizure disorders, sudden deaths, and mental illness, as these may be subtle manifestations of the condition affecting the patient at hand.

NEWBORN SCREENING (NBS)

Until the mid-2000s mandatory screening of newborns was highly variable state to state, with some screening as few as six conditions and others screening for dozens of conditions. In 2006, the American College of Medical Genetics and Genomics (ACMG) published a report recommending a standard panel of tests[1]. Today, a minimum of 31 core disorders are tested in all 50 states of the United States. The practitioner should be aware of when diseases were added to the NBS requirements in a particular state to avoid falsely assuming that a child with symptoms of an inborn error of metabolism underwent NBS. As time passes fewer and fewer patients under age 18 will have missed out on NBS. Newborn screening encompasses disorders that are not necessarily genetic, such as hypothyroidism, hearing loss, and congenital heart disease. These are beyond the scope of this text.

NBS: Collecting and reporting

The precise details of the timing of collection, method of collection, method of analysis, and reporting process vary from state to state and internationally. An excellent resource is http://www.babysfirsttest.org/, which compiles information for parents and professionals regarding the diseases screened, collection and reporting methods, and links to each state's NBS site.

The following are key and practical points to consider when examining results of NBS:

- Ideally, parents should be counseled about possible results from NBS at the time it is sent. This could reduce anxiety when screens return positive and perhaps increase parents' willingness to obtaining follow-up labs. In reality most parents are unaware that a complex screen was sent on their infant, in part due to the time required to provide counseling during the busy neonatal period, and also for fear that discussing the NBS will cause some parents anxiety such that they opt out of the screen, which should be firmly discouraged.

- The timing of blood spot collection is important to the interpretation of NBS results. Some metabolites require time after the separation of the baby from the placenta to accumulate to levels that will reliably flag on NBS. Phenylalanine—elevated in phenylketonuria—is one such metabolite. Most states accept samples from infants older than 12 hours of age.

- A sample can be collected earlier than a state's cutoff if the infant will be transfused, but a later sample should also be sent. Some states test enzymes present in red blood cells that will be falsely normal if the infant was transfused. Some states will test cord blood if no pretransfusion sample is available. It is worth becoming familiar with local policies.

- Responses to positive screens should be individualized based on the potential disorder, the degree of abnormality of the measured metabolite, the clinical status of then newborn, and the advice of a consulting specialist. Such responses include determining if the child needs to see a specialist, any dietary changes that might be necessary, and specific symptoms to monitor. Timely confirmatory testing is critical.

- For most metabolic conditions detected by NBS, while confirmatory testing is pending, the most important intervention is to avoid catabolism, which demands regular feeding (approximately every three hours, which most newborns do anyway) and a rapid response to any decreased feeding, change in mental status, or other concerning symptoms.

- In cases where the newborn is asymptomatic, the primary care provider is usually the most appropriate point person for the parents' questions until confirmatory test results return.

NBS: Unscreened children

Infants who did not have NBS performed in the immediate newborn period should undergo screening. However, the metabolite cutoffs for positive and negative screens are designed for newborns and thus may be more likely to yield both false-positive and false-negative results. Health care practitioners should be aware of the circumstances that might be associated with a child's having missed the newborn screen, including birth in a developing country or outside of a health care setting (e.g., home birth). For unscreened, asymptomatic older children (school age and physically/developmentally normal), the yield from performing screening is low and opinions vary as to its utility. In the case of an unscreened child *with symptoms* that could be consistent with a disorder on the NBS (including but not limited to any delay in development or any neurologic symptoms), testing must be guided by the phenotype and can include formal metabolic testing—rather than simply sending a newborn screen to the state—ideally in consultation with a specialist (Table 3-1).

NBS: Sensitivity and specificity

NBS programs are designed to be sensitive and because it is difficult to achieve a high positive predictive value (PPV) from a screen for rare diseases (see Appendix 7), the NBS therefore produces far more false-positives than false-negatives for most metabolic components of the screen. False-positives are probably the major downside to current NBS paradigms, and evidence exists that there can be lasting psychological consequences wherein parents never

Table 3-1. Tests to cover metabolic portion of NBS conditions in a symptomatic, older child.

Test	Notes
Acylcarnitine profile	Lab codes provided in Chapter 4
Free and total carnitine	Lab codes provided in Chapter 4
Plasma amino acid analysis	Lab codes provided in Chapter 4
Urine organic acid analysis	Lab codes provided in Chapter 4
Biotinidase activity	LabCorp: #402362 Mayo: BIOTS Quest: #70132
Thyroid studies	Consider if symptoms are consistent
Cystic fibrosis testing	Consider if symptoms are consistent
Galactosemia testing	Consider if symptoms are consistent

shake the idea that there is "something wrong" with their baby even if the child turns out to be perfectly healthy[2]. A primary care provider must balance the urgency of obtaining follow-up testing on newborns with positive screens with calming and supporting the family.

Talking to a family about a positive NBS

There are not enough metabolic specialists in the world to assure that every baby with a positive newborn screen is seen immediately in clinic. For this reason, the primary care practitioner is an essential first-line health care professional who interacts with the family. In most states, the primary care provider will be able to talk to a specialist by phone, and there is much information that should be communicated during that conversation. Table 3-2 is a checklist intended to assist the practitioner in obtaining the necessary information to help the family with its next steps.

> ### Key Point
>
> Newborn screening challenges primary care pediatricians to communicate with families and specialists, arrange testing, and monitor the baby, all the while minimizing the parents' anxiety.

Practice Point: Clinical Counseling

Warning: This is a sample conversation only and *will not* be applicable to all situations. Confirm all information with the state lab and/or assisting specialist. Always examine the baby and send confirmatory testing without delay. Newborns with any abnormal symptoms should be directed to the nearest emergency department and the assisting specialist must be notified.

Sample conversation with parents of an asymptomatic child with an abnormal newborn screen.

"As you may be aware, every child born in this state has a small amount of blood taken in the first few days of life which is sent to a lab to look for rare genetic conditions that can be treated better if detected early. I just spoke with the state and with a geneticist, and your son/daughter had a positive screen for _____, which is a rare genetic condition. Before I say anything more, I want you to understand that more babies have positive screens than actually have diseases, so there is a chance that your baby does not have that disorder. If your baby does have it he/she will be seen by a specialist to discuss therapies and answer your questions. But we need to send some more lab work to know for sure.

Let me ask you, is your baby eating well, and awake and alert between naps?

I would like to see your baby as soon as possible (ideally today). Please bring your baby to _____ lab today (if at all possible), to have the labs drawn. It will take _____ days/weeks to get results, and I will let you know as soon as I receive them. Please call me immediately or go to an emergency room if your baby won't eat, seems unusually sleepy, or is acting in a way that concerns you. The specialist in this case *did/didn't* recommend a change in your baby's diet. I'll check in with you periodically while we wait.

I know this is stressful, but I am here to answer your questions until we get the results back. Remember that many babies with positive screens are *just fine*; but to be safe we need to do further testing."

	Table 3-2. Checklist to assist practitioners in helping a family with a positive newborn screening test.
☐	Obtain the exact name of the disease or diseases indicated by the screen[a].
☐	Check whether the abnormal lab value gives the specialist any insight into the likelihood that this is a true or false positive[b].
☐	Find out exactly what lab tests will be necessary to confirm or rule out the diagnosis.
☐	Find out if it matters when the lab is sent relative to when the baby eats.
☐	Learn what signs or symptoms should be monitored in the newborn and how frequently until confirmatory results return.
☐	Obtain an estimate of how long it will take to receive follow-up test results, and how they will be communicated.

[a]Be aware that sometimes an abnormal metabolite can be observed in more than one disorder, and further testing will be necessary to clarify the precise diagnosis, if one exists.
[b]For some metabolic diseases, the degree of deviation from normal of the abnormal metabolite can correlate with the probability of its being a true positive. Any child with a value outside the state's cutoff must receive prompt follow-up testing, but given that part of the role of the primary provider is to calm and educate the parents, it can be helpful to know if, in the experience of the consulting specialist, a particular child's lab is more or less likely to be confirmed as a true positive.

NBS: ACMG ACTion (ACT) Sheets

The ACMG has created educational resources for physicians and other providers who need information about NBS results and subsequent management. These are excellent references and we encourage all who care for newborns to review them. However, because the evidence for each particular test or intervention is limited and complex, many geneticists deviate somewhat from the ACT Sheets. It is best to follow the advice of the consulting geneticist.[1]

Resolving newborn screen cases

Many positive newborn screens are false-positives and the child does not require any additional evaluation after confirmatory testing returns negative. In cases where the child is confirmed to be positive a prompt referral should be made to a specialist, if one is not already involved. For a few disorders such as glutaric acidemia type I (GA1) and very-long chain acyl-CoA dehydrogenase deficiency (VLCADD), metabolite levels may be abnormal only transiently in the newborn period and then normalize on confirmatory testing even if the disorder is present. Practices vary in these situations. Some

[1] https://www.acmg.net/ACMG/Publications/ACT_Sheets_and_Confirmatory_Algorithms/NBS_ACT_Sheets_and_Algorithm_Table/ACMG/Publications/ACT_Sheets_and_Confirmatory_Algorithms/NBS_ACT_Sheets_and_Algorithms_Table.aspx?hkey=e2c16055-8cdc-4b22-a53b-b863622007c0

specialists will obtain gene sequencing in all cases, while others only seek sequencing in select cases.

For other disorders such as short-chain acyl-CoA dehydrogenase deficiency (SCADD) and 3-methylcrotonyl-CoA carboxylase deficiency (3-MCC) evidence is mounting that individuals with these biochemical defects are healthy without any therapy for the disorder. Some countries and states have removed these conditions from screening but many have not and practices still vary in terms of the types of treatments recommended. Finally, many diseases on the newborn screen have intermediate forms, most notably phenylketonuria and galactosemia. Patients have milder defects in the involved enzymes and thus do not have the classic disorders but still may require monitoring.

The future of newborn screening

The original purpose of NBS was to identify diseases that might be, at least to some degree, treatable if recognized before the onset of symptoms. For example, children identified with severe combined immunodeficiency (SCID) tolerate bone marrow transplantation (which can be curative) much better if they are not already suffering from chronic infections[3]. The ACMG recommends that disorders considered for NBS possess, at a minimum, the following characteristics:

1. The disease can be identified in the first days of life.
2. The test is appropriately sensitive and specific.
3. There are benefits to early detection.

These characteristics are broadly applicable to any screening program, as outlined by Wilson and Junger in 1968. All of these basic criteria are being challenged by both the rapid development of sequence-based diagnostics and advocacy around certain diseases, and both primary practitioners and the lay public will have to become more informed to navigate an upcoming onslaught of new and complex options for genetic screening in newborns.

Already private labs have begun to offer NBS products to doctors and even direct to consumers (e.g., https://www.babygenes.net/). These sequencing technologies cover current NBS conditions and also other childhood-onset genetic diseases. Geneticists expect that sequence-based screening will eventually replace metabolite testing, but "upgrading" to sequence-based NBS will not be simple. The following are important challenges:

- As of today, the inability to interpret many variants in genes causing diseases on today's newborn screens limits the utility of sequencing as the primary newborn screen. Metabolite testing looks at the actual biochemical phenotype and therefore is immune to the challenge of classifying variants as benign or pathogenic (see Appendix 6 for a discussion of variant interpretation). Sequence-based screens probably have an excellent negative predictive value (NPV) to rule out a disorder when no variants are found, but cannot yet replace metabolite-based screening without further research.

- Many disorders tested by sequence-based panels are untreatable. Not all families will want to know this type of information.

- Some recessive disorders on sequence-based panels actually can cause symptoms in the carrier parent(s). These include X-linked adrenoleukodystrophy, Gaucher disease, and Fragile X. Parents should be made aware that testing their newborn may unexpectedly reveal information about their own health.

- Given that >99% of newborns do not have a disease on current state NBS panels, it may be difficult to justify the added cost of sequencing all newborns until the price of sequencing decreases and there is evidence of benefit from this additional screening. Sequencing for symptomatic newborns or those with positive screens may be more appropriate in the near-term.

- Newborn screening traditionally has been hailed as a success story of early diagnosis. With ongoing advancements in carrier screening and prenatal diagnosis, should we not begin to view detecting a disease in a newborn as too late? If parents are undergoing carrier screening for the same conditions (see Chapter 1), how can this information be used to maximize reproductive options, and then be incorporated into the child's newborn screen to reduce redundancy?

It is inevitable that more and more genetic diseases will be added to NBS, and because more therapies currently are available, metabolic disorders will be at the forefront for new screening panels. Some diseases will be part of state-mandated screens while others will be optionally available to parents who can afford them. While the U.S. Food and Drug Administration (FDA) is moving to regulate these tests, instilling some manner of uniformity and predictability (see Appendix 7), such regulation will be an ongoing and iterative process. There are insufficient metabolic specialists to be the first line in the management of positive results from these new screens. Primary practitioners will need to know how to approach patients with positive screens. This will include (1) a basic familiarity with the screening tests and covered diseases, (2) a familiarity with follow-up testing and how to order it, and (3) a relationship with the appropriate specialists to seek guidance and make referrals when needed.

For symptomatic newborns or children, some sequencing panels are available (e.g., for common conditions, or broad neurologic conditions) with rapid turnaround, often <2 weeks (e.g., babygenes mentioned above). The proper place of such tests in the diagnosis of newborns is difficult to assess. On one hand, these panels are thoughtfully designed and screen for many more disorders than traditional metabolic testing in a slightly longer timeframe compared to biochemical tests (and much faster than typical whole-exome sequencing (WES), though this is changing). They can be a useful addition to the genetic toolbox. On the other hand, they are considerably more expensive than metabolic testing or targeted gene testing and are not nearly as complete as WES. Anecdotally, many clinical geneticists feel that they could diagnose most children more efficiently than a one-size-fits-all gene panel, but this claim is unproven, as is any claim that a particular sequencing test performs better than clinical judgment. Newborn disease panels are particularly attractive in settings where a trained geneticist is unavailable, but the advisability of developing large gene panels over simply improving access to trained geneticists is worthy of consideration.

THE DYSMORPHIC CHILD

The general practitioner can contribute substantially to the evaluation and diagnosis of children with birth defects and dysmorphic features and help a family know what to expect when they are evaluated by a specialist.

Define the phenotype

As humans, we are programmed to look at faces, and dysmorphic facial features are often the most prominent. However, a thorough evaluation requires the assessment of the whole body, inside and out, and the general practitioner can accomplish a great deal of this evaluation! An introduction to this approach is given below.

Major dysmorphic features

Dysmorphic features can be conceptually divided into major and minor features. Major features are either severe (e.g., congenital cardiac malformation) or unusual (e.g., syndactyly). Major features generally serve as a starting point to *generate* a differential diagnosis. One of the most common major features is developmental delay, and a careful determination of developmental milestones (gross and fine motor, social, language) is absolutely essential in any child with a suspected genetic syndrome.

A complete physical exam, including careful evaluation of the eyes, oral cavity, hands, and genitals, comprises the first step of a dysmorphology exam. Typical studies to identify internal malformations include: brain imaging (MRI or ultrasound), abdominal and renal ultrasound, skeletal survey to visualize the long bones and vertebrae, ophthalmologic examination, and echocardiography. Which of these studies should be obtained in a given patient, and in what order, must be guided by the urgency with which a diagnosis is needed, the extent and location(s) of external malformations, consultation with an expert, and the differential diagnosis under consideration.

> **Key Point**
>
> It is appropriate to be sure that a child's phenotype (the summation of historical, physical, laboratory, and imaging findings) is as complete as possible before embarking on genetic testing.
>
> Even with sophisticated genomic testing, the genotype must match the phenotype to establish a diagnosis, which of course requires a defined phenotype.

Conducting such an evaluation in an efficient and cost-effective manner can be challenging. For example, a congenital heart anomaly represents the type of malformation most likely to kill a newborn if it is not identified promptly. On the other hand, pediatric echocardiography can be difficult to obtain in some localities. It is therefore crucial that a general practitioner perform a thorough cardiac evaluation (4-limb blood pressures, palpation of distal pulses, pre and postductal oxygen saturation, chest auscultation) in any newborn with dysmorphic features to inform the urgency of obtaining echocardiography. As a child ages, grows, and feeds well, a congenital cardiac malformation becomes less likely, though echocardiography may still be appropriate as part of an evaluation.

Minor dysmorphic features

The purpose of identifying minor features serves to *narrow* the differential diagnosis generated by the major feature(s). The formation of every part of the body is subject to countless variations, and some are more likely to be associated with genetic disease than others. Standardized terms have been developed to describe the visible body (http://elementsofmorphology.nih .gov/). Low-set ears, single palmar creases, or slanting palpebral fissures are among the more recognized minor dysmorphic features. Generally, the co-occurrence of many minor dysmorphic features increases the likelihood of the presence of a major feature and an underlying genetic disorder. It must be stressed that these minor features do not constitute evidence of a genetic disease in and of themselves, and minor features are present in some proportion of healthy individuals and can be more frequent in some ethnic groups.

Trisomy 21 (Down syndrome)

Trisomy 21 is possibly the most common genetic condition encountered by primary pediatrics professionals, and thus some discussion is warranted here.

First, a superb review of the recommended screening and therapies for individuals with Trisomy 21 at any age is available and should be familiar to anyone who cares for children[4].

Screening for trisomies during pregnancy is common (see Chapter 2) and thus many families are aware that their child has a trisomy even before birth. A familiarity with the diagnosis and course of Trisomy 21 is important to assist these families at every stage. It is useful to know that while the risk of Trisomy 21 does increase with maternal age, about 80% of babies with Trisomy 21 are born to women younger than 35 years. There are several excellent resources for families with children with Trisomy 21 (see Appendix 11 for web resources).

In addition to the recommended screening tests detailed in the reference above, another important role of the practitioner in the management of Trisomy 21 is to confirm the diagnosis and that it does not result from a translocation. Most Trisomy 21 is de novo, but about 3% of Trisomy 21 is caused by an inherited translocation where a parent could have a copy of chromosome 21 stuck to another chromosome. In this scenario, the risk of future children also having Trisomy 21 can be very high, and thus these cases must be identified to provide accurate reproductive counseling to the parents.

If a primary care practitioner feels comfortable caring for a patient with Trisomy 21 there is no need for an urgent referral to a geneticist. Clinical geneticists' main role is to assist the primary care provider in following the recommended screening and to answer questions when unusual symptoms or concerns arise. Establishing a relationship between a family and a geneticist should any such questions arise is generally a sound strategy.

What happens when a dysmorphic child is seen by a geneticist?

A geneticist uses two processes when evaluating a new patient: diagnostic testing and screening. If the child's features and history are consistent with a diagnosis recognized by the geneticist, he or she may proceed with specific diagnostic testing of individual genes. However, as is often the case, if the features are not entirely classic for a single disorder, the geneticist will opt to send screening tests that look for many disorders at once. The geneticist will often combine diagnostic and screening tests either simultaneously or sequentially depending on the differential diagnosis and suspected yield of each test. Diagnostic tests are specific to each of thousands of disorders and cannot be listed here. The most commonly used screening tests are given below.

Chromosomal microarray analysis: As discussed in detail in Appendix 2, microarray analysis is currently the most available genome-wide screening test, and is often the initial screen for a child with unusual or complex medical complaints. It is an appropriate first-line test in children with developmental delay, autism, and/or congenital anomalies[5]. In common situations, such as a prolonged wait to see a geneticist or if the family is unable to travel to a specialist, it is appropriate for a nongeneticist practitioner to order an array. Nearly all major diagnostics laboratories perform array studies, and the reader is directed to Appendix 2 to understand better the strengths and limitations of the test. Involving a geneticist, even remotely, in the interpretation of an array result is recommended.

Karyotype: Karyotypes remain important tests in the genetics armamentarium and can provide information that an array cannot (see Appendix 2), but as an initial screening test for many suspected genetic conditions the karyotype has essentially been replaced by array technologies. Karyotypes are now primarily used in specific scenarios when a large chromosomal rearrangement or aneuploidy is suspected. In general, do not order a karyotype as a first-line screening test unless large chromosomal changes are implicated in the phenotype in question (e.g., ambiguous genitalia, features of Down syndrome, recurrent miscarriages), or after speaking with a specialist.

Whole-genome/exome sequencing: A discussion of whole-genome/exome sequencing can be found in Chapter 5[6].

Metabolic screening: Even for children with normal newborn screens, testing for inborn errors of metabolism (IEMs) may be indicated, and are discussed in more detail in Chapters 4 and 5. Most of these tests are not familiar to the nongeneticist, but can be ordered pending a visit to a specialist to speed the diagnostic evaluation.

THE FUTURE AND ETHICS OF NEWBORN GENETICS

The advent of genome-wide screening technologies such as microarrays and WES has brought about a revolution in the diagnosis of birth defects and other genetic syndromes. Today, these tests still are ordered primarily by specialists after an exam and initial evaluation, but most professional geneticists expect that these tests will become increasingly affordable and available, and thus will be ordered increasingly early in the diagnostic process, possibly even before a specialist is involved. Eventually whole-genome analyses will be employed for everyone at birth in anticipation of future health needs. Much work remains to be done before this can occur effectively and efficiently.

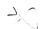

> **Key Point**
>
> The exploding yields of advanced genetic tests, combined with limited access to genetics specialists, are likely to place nongeneticist practitioners increasingly in a position where they may consider ordering complex genomic tests before a specialist can be formally involved.

As discussed, the phenotypic evaluation (history/physical/lab/imaging information) of a patient can be expensive and invasive. As the proverbial cart is increasingly placed before the genetic horse, if you will, with more extensive sequencing and NBS, medicine runs the risk of subjecting newborns and children to medical workups based on unclear findings on genomic tests. For example, if a seemingly normal newborn has a variant in a gene known to be associated with agenesis of the corpus callosum, would it be appropriate to sedate the infant for a brain MRI? Would it be better to wait and see if development proceeds normally, and intervene only if delay becomes apparent? To provide truly evidence-based care, studies will be required that compare outcomes from patients who have been managed by different approaches. Few such studies exist today. When it comes to genomic medicine, general practitioners and geneticists must navigate these uncharted seas by employing sound judgment, expert consultation, and a collaborative approach with the patients and families.

Ethics

In most developed countries, NBS is mandatory and parents must opt-out if they do not desire screening. Whenever a medical procedure (e.g., vaccines) is required that affects a minor it is important to remember that the patient cannot consent, placing a burden on the medical system and parents to be sure the test is substantially in the best interest of the child. By and large this is the case with NBS paradigms, but it can become easy to go too far, for example:

- Adding untreatable diseases such as lysosomal storage disorders. This may avoid a diagnostic odyssey in some patients, but will not improve the final outcome until therapies are developed.
- Screening genes with low penetrance or adult age of onset. Doing so may violate the future-adult's autonomy (see Appendix 9).
- Screening for conditions that cannot be adequately ruled in or out by subsequent testing. Doing so places the child in a perpetual state of limbo, waiting for symptoms to develop.

A publication on Krabbe disease screening in New York highlights these challenges[7]. The screen had a PPV of 1.4%, and of the four infants who underwent bone marrow transplantation to attempt to prevent disease progression, two died from complications of the transplant. Many more infants were left in a state of uncertainty because they had reduced enzyme function but it was not possible to determine if they would ever progress to be symptomatic. Screening for new disorders will continue to combine the voices of patient advocacy groups, scientists/physicians, and policy makers and will be fascinating to follow.

Most IEMs are recessive or X-linked, meaning that the causative mutations were already present in the parents before the child was conceived. As more and more individuals learn their carrier status due to advances in sequencing and genome interpretation, one might imagine that, with the exception of couples who consciously do not desire preconception testing, NBS could one day be considered a second-line means to a diagnosis.

Practice Point: Clinical Scenario 1

A premature newborn who has been on total parenteral nutrition (TPN) for several weeks receives a positive newborn screen for argininemia, a urea cycle defect, due to elevated arginine on the screen.

Points to consider:

1. How can one best inform the parents of this result without alarming them?
2. Who could be of assistance in arranging for follow-up testing? What metabolic tests would make sense?
3. While follow-up tests are pending, if the baby became neurologically unstable and the neonatologist wished to determine if argininemia could be contributing, what rapidly available test(s) could be sent?

Practice Point: Clinical Scenario 2

Parents of a dysmorphic infant want to know if whole-exome sequencing (WES) is the obvious first test for their infant.

Important points to make to the family are the following:

1. Whole-exome sequencing has revolutionized the diagnosis of rare diseases and may indeed yield a diagnosis for their child, but . . .

2. Currently WES is expensive and takes several months to return results. Waiting for insurance approval and processing may delay diagnosis if a more available test would have sufficed.

3. WES is not the ideal test for detecting copy number variations, trinucleotide repeats, methylation abnormalities, translocations, and other genomic alterations and is therefore not a complete test.

4. WES can return unexpected results that may lead down diagnostic rabbit holes. Such findings may be acceptable in pursuit of a diagnosis, but should be weighed before ordering WES.

5. There is no perfect test that is always the best first test for children with suspected rare diseases. Such children often undergo several rounds of testing before receiving a diagnosis.

REFERENCES

1. American College of Medical Genetics Newborn Screening Expert G. Newborn screening: toward a uniform screening panel and system—executive summary. *Pediatrics*. 2006;117 (5 pt 2):S296-S307. doi:10.1542/peds.2005-2633I.

2. Hewlett J, Waisbren SE. A review of the psychosocial effects of false-positive results on parents and current communication practices in newborn screening. *J Inherit Metab Dis*. 2006;29(5):677-682. doi:10.1007/s10545-006-0381-1.

3. Pai SY, Logan BR, Griffith LM, et al. Transplantation outcomes for severe combined immunodeficiency, 2000-2009. *N Engl J Med*. 2014;371(5):434-446. doi:10.1056/NEJMoa1401177.

4. Bull MJ, Committee on G. Health supervision for children with Down syndrome. *Pediatrics*. 2011;128(2):393-406. doi:10.1542/peds.2011-1605.

5. Manning M, Hudgins L, Professional P, Guidelines C. Array-based technology and recommendations for utilization in medical genetics practice for detection of chromosomal abnormalities. *Genet Med*. 2010;12(11):742-745. doi:10.1097/GIM.0b013e3181f8baad.

6. Retterer K, Juusola J, Cho MT, et al. Clinical application of whole-exome sequencing across clinical indications. *Genet Med*. 2015. doi:10.1038/gim.2015.148.

7. Orsini JJ, Kay DM, Saavedra-Matiz CA, et al. Newborn screening for Krabbe disease in New York State: the first eight years' experience. *Genet Med*. 2016. doi:10.1038/gim.2015.211.

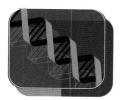

CHAPTER 4

Emergency Medic
Metabolic Disease

The crucial recognition that an Inborn Error of Metabolism (IEM) is at play often comes from a nongeneticist practitioner. Rather than serve as a textbook of the many biochemical pathways affected in IEMs, this section is intended as a general and practical overview to facilitate the initial recognition and early management of a suspected metabolic crisis and provide an introduction to the most common diagnostic and management strategies. The detailed diagnosis of IEMs, interpretation of complex biochemical labs, and the nuanced management of these patients is the purview of the specialist and therefore this section cannot replace timely consultation with a specialist should such a situation arise. Biochemical genetics is a subfield of Medical Genetics and physicians who specialize in this field are available around the world. Because of the rarity of IEMs, involvement of this type of specialist is often inevitable for diagnosis and management. Illnesses caused by IEMs that present more subtly (e.g., as developmental delay) are discussed in Chapter 5.

THE METABOLIC CRISIS

Table 4-1 provides a simplified association between diseases and metabolic findings that can present in crisis. Symptoms of an acute metabolic crisis often include a combination of altered mental status, seizures, organ dysfunction (particularly liver), rhabdomyolysis, or heart failure (potentially involving cardiomyopathy). Signs can include altered respiration (either tachypnea or bradypnea), an unusual odor, hepatomegaly, abnormal behavior or even psychotic symptoms, jaundice and other evidence of acute liver disease. Abnormalities detectable on routine laboratory studies can include acidosis (typically with an anion gap), hyperammonemia, elevated blood lactate, hypo- or hyperglycemia, or other electrolyte disturbances. Abnormalities in sodium and potassium may point to adrenal or other endocrine dysfunction. The challenge for the practitioner first is to consider a metabolic disturbance in the differential

> **Key Point**
>
> Most symptomatic patients with inherited metabolic diseases will first present to a pediatrician, neonatologist, or emergency medicine physician.

> **Key Point**
>
> **Essential** labs whenever a metabolic disorder is suspected:
>
> - Complete metabolic panel (Na, K, Cl, CO_2, BUN, creatinine, glucose, AST, ALT, alkaline phosphatase and/or GGT, direct/indirect bilirubin, protein, albumin, Ca, Mg, Phos)
> - Urinalysis (glucose, ketones, nitrite, leukocyte esterase, pH)
> - Blood gas (capillary or venous is acceptable)
> - Creatine kinase (noncardiac isoform)
> - Ammonia
> - Lactate
>
> Strongly consider:
>
> - CBC with differential
> - Homocysteine

Table 4-1. Presenting findings during metabolic crisis and some associated diseases.

Presenting finding(s)	Typical metabolic disease category
Hyperammonemia alone	Urea cycle defect
Hyperammonemia with anion gap acidosis	Organic acid disorders
Hyperammonemia with hypoglycemia	Fatty acid oxidation disorders Organic acid disorders
Hypoglycemia	Fatty acid oxidation disorder (esp. without ketosis) Glycogen storage disease (often with hepatomegaly) Hyperinsulinemia
Hypoglycemia with anion gap acidosis	Organic acid disorders
Lactic acidosis	Mitochondrial disease Pyruvate dehydrogenase deficiency Glycogen storage disease Disorders of gluconeogenesis Variety of other metabolic disorders
Rhabdomyolysis	Fatty acid oxidation disorder
Encephalopathy with few lab findings	Maple Syrup Urine Disease

diagnosis, and then to identify which signs, symptoms, and laboratory studies support this conclusion to guide initial management. While it may seem preferable to delay sending advanced metabolic studies until a specialist can consult, the practitioner should be familiar with and comfortable sending advanced metabolic screens because delaying testing delays a diagnosis. Test interpretation should be done in consultation with a qualified geneticist, but the testing itself need not be postponed for a specialist.

Some situations particularly demand that an IEM be explored. These include any acute illness in a newborn, any unexplained altered mental status in a child, and any condition that seems specifically to affect energy-intensive tissues, such as brain, liver, and muscle/heart and is not explained by more common diagnoses such as trauma or infection.

Essential basic laboratory studies when an IEM is being considered include a measurement of blood pH, glucose, urinalysis, serum (and sometimes urine) electrolytes with calculation of the anion gap, "liver function tests," lactate, and ammonia. Measuring urine glucose and reducing substances can be a rapid means to diagnose galactosemia if it is suspected but cannot definitively be ruled out. Creatine kinase (noncardiac isoform) levels can assist in identifying rhabdomyolysis or other conditions causing muscle breakdown. Abnormalities in any of these tests can be caused by nongenetic conditions, which must also be considered and addressed. Most modern hospitals are able to process the above tests rapidly. Caution must be exercised in the collection of the lactate and ammonia samples, as spuriously elevated values may be caused by poor collection technique (use of a tourniquet, trauma at the puncture site, incorrect collection tube, failure to immediately cool and process the samples). Potassium levels may be artificially elevated in hemolyzed samples. Capillary blood samples are not reliable for measuring lactate or ammonia and produce falsely elevated results.

Central themes

A practitioner dealing with a suspected IEM should note the following when undertaking initial evaluation and management:

1. Laboratory studies are needed to make a diagnosis. This means that the treating physician must be sure these studies are sent, and sent correctly. Critically, some labs will only return diagnostic results during a crisis and cannot wait until transfer to a specialty center or for outpatient follow up. The more data that is gathered during an acute episode, the more likely an IEM can be considered lower on the differential diagnosis, or that a specialist can diagnose an IEM efficiently. Which tests to send are suggested below, but a specialist should ideally be consulted, even by phone.

2. Catabolism is bad. Starvation, or reduced caloric intake in the setting of increased demand (e.g., from infection, trauma, or surgery), is a major precipitating factor for many metabolic crises. Provision of abundant carbohydrate in the form of IV dextrose (10% at 1.5 × maintenance fluid requirements) is a sound initial management strategy for nearly all suspected IEMs and can be instituted while laboratory studies and expert consultation is pending.

3. A well-appearing patient with an IEM can deteriorate rapidly, and the typical 6th sense of a trained pediatrician as to which children are sick can be falsely reassuring. Put simply, the homeostatic mechanisms that keep healthy children healthy don't work in patients with an IEM and cannot necessarily be relied upon.

The following sections will consider the initial management of several common presentations of metabolic crises.

ANION GAP METABOLIC ACIDOSIS

Initial evaluation

In the case of an elevated anion gap, the first step is to determine the identity of the abnormally elevated anion. The most common endogenous anions are lactate and ketones. Lactate can be measured rapidly in most hospitals.

By converting the lactate level and anion gap to be expressed in the same units, one can determine if the elevation in lactate is sufficient to explain the anion gap. Ketones may be quickly but crudely estimated by urine dipstick. Massive urinary ketones in the setting of an anion gap acidosis suggest the presence of a ketoacidosis which may or may not be physiologic (severe ketosis is less likely to be physiologic in a newborn). The differential diagnosis for ketoacidosis is broad and can include severe catabolism of any cause (starvation, infection, injury), diabetic ketoacidosis, as well as IEMs. Serum glucose measurement should be obtained to evaluate for diabetic ketoacidosis.

The differential diagnosis of lactic acidosis is broad and can include sepsis, heart disease, liver dysfunction, hypoxia, trauma, carbon monoxide poisoning, severe anemia, toxic ingestion, any process causing poor perfusion systemically or to any organ, as well as numerous IEMs. Because the former causes of lactic acidosis are far more common than IEMs, these considerations should be addressed most urgently. In addition to the advanced metabolic studies recommended below, should an IEM be suspected in the setting of a lactic acidosis, the possibility of a mitochondrial disease can be partially addressed by sending a repeat lactate level with a simultaneous pyruvate level. The pyruvate level is only interpretable in the setting of elevated lactate, and thus cannot wait until the patient has recovered. The pyruvate sample must also be frozen shortly after being drawn. Most hospitals do not process this laboratory as rapidly as lactate and several days may be required to receive results. Of course, pyruvate measurement is not useful in situations when the lactic acidosis is not caused by an IEM.

If an anion gap exists without sufficiently elevated lactate or ketones to account for the elevation, then the source of the anion requires more detailed investigation. Toxin ingestions must be considered as well as renal dysfunction. Unless an explanation is apparent for the gap acidosis, more advanced metabolic testing is indicated at this point (see table below for ordering details).

- Plasma total and free carnitine
- Plasma acyl-carnitine profile
- Plasma amino acid analysis
- Urine organic acid analysis

These metabolic screening laboratories will detect many IEMs that cause an acute anion gap acidosis. Broadly, these are the fundamental first-line metabolic screening labs for any patient with a suspected IEM. In most hospitals these are sent to a specialty lab and results are not available immediately, but these are inexpensive tests, can be very valuable to the future workup of the patient, and should be sent whenever the cause of a metabolic acidosis is not clear. As will be discussed below, diagnostic metabolites may only be elevated in the setting of an acute crisis and therefore testing should not wait until the patient is recovering. Further, if the patient continues to worsen, disease-targeted therapy will be impossible without a metabolic diagnosis. Providers who might encounter patients in acute metabolic crises should feel empowered to order these tests, but of course expert consultation is often appropriate as well.

Management

Management of a lactic acidosis should begin with supportive care aimed at ensuring adequate perfusion (e.g., providing saline boluses, monitoring blood pressure) and identifying any potential nongenetic causes or exacerbating factors that would increase energy demand or decrease oxygenation and/or perfusion. Inborn causes of lactic acidosis can involve many different forms of mitochondrial dysfunction, as well as defects in gluconeogenesis or glycogen storage (more likely if the lactic acidosis is accompanied by hypoglycemia). Mitochondrial diseases are major hereditary causes of lactic acidosis, but in general highly effective therapies are lacking. Vitamin cocktails are sometimes attempted, and consultation with a specialist would be appropriate if this intervention is being considered.

Ketogenesis occurs predominantly in the liver and is regulated primarily by insulin. Therefore, providing abundant carbohydrate (most urgently in the form of IV dextrose, at least 10% dextrose at 1.5 × maintenance fluid requirements) provides calories to address catabolism as well as stimulates endogenous insulin secretion that in turn shuts off ketosis. In severe cases of ketoacidosis, exogenous insulin may need to be supplied to stop ketosis effectively. Administration of insulin with glucose in the setting of severe ketoacidosis, even in a nondiabetic, is acceptable management in the appropriate intensive care setting with adequate monitoring of blood glucose to prevent hypoglycemia.

Even if the anion cannot be identified with standard lab tests, an aggressive glucose infusion to address catabolism is an excellent starting point. Bicarbonate can be administered if the acidosis is extreme, and dialysis may be rarely required.

HYPOGLYCEMIA

The differential diagnosis of hypoglycemia in a child is also lengthy and can involve not only IEMs, but also endocrine or hepatic dysfunction, or simply a state of severe stress such as infection or trauma. Many of these causes are beyond the scope of this handbook of genetics. Nevertheless, the essential laboratory studies indicated at the beginning of this chapter, particularly if drawn immediately at the time hypoglycemia is noted, can be useful in pointing the diagnostic compass toward or away from a genetic cause. If possible, ordering advanced metabolic studies listed in the table at the end of the chapter can also be helpful, particularly in a child with recurrent hypoglycemia, though follow-up with a specialist would be prudent as well. Measurement of blood insulin, cortisol, and growth hormone levels during hypoglycemia are important components of the endocrine workup. Palpation of an enlarged liver can suggest some types of glycogen storage disease.

HYPERAMMONEMIA

Hyperammonemia is a true medical emergency. In a child with open cranial sutures, the ensuing cerebral edema is not lethal but highly neurotoxic. The risk of developmental delay after a single episode of severe hyperammonemia is exceedingly high, highlighting the need for rapid action. In an older child or adult, cerebral edema due to hyperammonemia can cause herniation and death. Disorders that cause hyperammonemia can present at any age and there is a robust literature on first-time adult presentations.

Ammonia comes from two sources: breakdown of dietary protein, and breakdown of endogenous protein. Whenever dietary protein exceeds anabolic needs (which is the case in nearly anyone eating a normal diet) the remainder is broken down for energy, releasing ammonia. In a catabolic state (e.g., starvation, infection, glucocorticoid therapy), endogenous protein is broken down, again releasing ammonia. Normally, ammonia is converted to urea rapidly, primarily in the liver, and excreted. In patients with urea cycle defects, or a number of other IEMs that indirectly impact the urea cycle, ammonia accumulates in the blood. The mechanisms of toxicity of ammonia are incompletely understood, but the primary target organ is the brain. Symptoms of hyperammonemia include altered mental status ranging from lethargy to coma, hyperventilation (often with alkalosis) progressing to apnea, seizures, and sometimes an odor. Hyperammonemia is on the differential diagnosis for unexplained tachypnea in an infant.

As is the case with any clinical presentation or lab abnormality, IEMs are not alone on the differential diagnosis. The most common nongenetic cause of hyperammonemia is liver failure from any cause. Importantly, hyperammonemia due to an IEM is managed differently from that seen in chronic liver disease, as described below.

Initial evaluation

Whenever a metabolic process is suspected, the essential labs above must be sent. A number of genetic defects can cause hyperammonemia and a specific diagnosis cannot be reached without advanced testing. Total and free carnitine, an acyl-carnitine profile, urine organic acids, and plasma amino acids must be sent. One additional lab to be aware of is urine orotic acid, which should be sent in any case of unexplained hyperammonemia.

Mild hyperammonemia can be diagnostically challenging as causes are varied, but a symptomatic patient without a clear explanation for the hyperammonemia, particularly an infant or child, should be treated aggressively, at least with a dextrose infusion and close monitoring of ammonia. Recommended interventions at a given ammonia level are difficult to pinpoint because much depends on the clinical context and trend in ammonia. Generally, an ammonia level greater than 200 μM immediately should raise suspicion for an IEM, with initiation of a dextrose infusion, temporary reduction of protein intake, and plans to provide ammonia scavenging agents (see the section Management below).

Management

Treatment of hyperammonemia involves two approaches: reducing the breakdown of protein and removing ammonia from the body.

Because dietary protein can be broken down into ammonia, it is critical that all dietary protein intake be temporarily reduced or stopped. As hyperammonemic patients often are critically ill, they usually are highly catabolic and thus the breakdown of endogenous protein also contributes to the total ammonia load. As some disorders of fatty acid oxidation also can lead to hyperammonemia, withholding fat is an appropriate initial maneuver until a fatty acid oxidation defect can be ruled out. Providing abundant calories in the form of IV dextrose (10% dextrose at 1.5 × maintenance fluid requirements) provides calories and can reverse catabolism in the short term. Identifying and treating other causes of catabolism (e.g., infection) is essential.

No one can live without taking in protein, and a patient will become protein deficient and start breaking down endogenous protein if all dietary protein is withheld for more than 1–2 days, or even sooner, depending on the age of the patient. Therefore, prolonged withholding of dietary protein is impossible. After stabilizing the patient and instituting an aggressive IV dextrose infusion, resumption of some protein intake must be undertaken with the advice of a qualified metabolic specialist or dietician, even if a diagnosis has not yet been reached.

Hyperammonemia in a patient with chronic liver disease generally is treated by administering lactulose and neomycin. Lactulose acts by acidifying the colon and trapping protonated ammonia (ammonium) in the gut where it is excreted. This is appropriate when the liver is generally dysfunctional and a chronic alternative route for ammonia elimination must be utilized. However, lactulose is *not* the preferred method to treat hyperammonemia due to an IEM. It is too inefficient, and the ensuing diarrhea can cause dehydration that, in a child, only would worsen the situation. Instead, ammonia scavenging agents (oral sodium phenylbutyrate (BuPhenyl) or IV sodium benzoate/sodium phenylacetate (Ammonul)) are recommended. These agents remove ammonia from nitrogen-containing amino acids in the body (glutamine, glycine) and then free ammonia is used to reform the amino acids, thus clearing ammonia. These drugs often only are available at specialized centers and should be managed by a specialist. Access to these medications for patients with more than mild hyperammonemia is a common reason to transfer the patient to a specialty center.

If hyperammonemia is severe (>400 μM, though practices vary), the most rapid way to remove ammonia is hemodialysis. Because ammonia distributes in all tissues, rapid removal of ammonia from the blood by dialysis may be followed by a rebound as ammonia redistributes from the tissues; the clinician should be prepared for this and not discontinue dialysis prematurely.

The general practitioner would not be expected to interpret the results of the more advanced metabolic studies mentioned in Table 4-2, but must be prepared to send the studies when a patient is in crisis. Importantly, the time required for results to return from such tests varies widely depending on the lab, but is rarely less than two days, necessitating

Key Point

The value of promptly sending metabolic testing during an acute presentation cannot be overstated. A specialist should still be consulted, at least by phone, if possible.

Table 4-2. Advanced metabolic laboratory studies to be sent in any likely metabolic emergency.

Test	Code	Notes
Acyl-carnitine profile, plasma	Quest #14531 LabCorp #070228 ARUP #0040033	Blood, about 1 mL, sodium heparin tube, freeze plasma at −20°C
Total and free carnitine, plasma	Quest #70107 LabCorp #706500 ARUP #0080068	Blood, about 1 mL, sodium heparin tube, freeze plasma at −20°C
Amino acid profile, quantitative, plasma	Quest #varies by region Labcorp #700068 ARUP #2009389	Blood, about 1 mL, heparin tube, freeze plasma at −20°C
Organic acids, qualitative, urine	LabCorp #716720 ARUP #0098389 Quest #90404	>5 mL, urine cup no preservatives, freeze at −20°C
Orotic acid, urine	LabCorp #007010 ARUP #0092458 Quest #11061 (may vary by region)	Send only for unexplained hyperammonemia

Disclaimer: These test codes are provided for reference only; no endorsement is made of any diagnostic company. As test codes are subject to change, confirm that the code matches the description before ordering. Blood volumes, tube type, and storage may vary by diagnostic lab. Confirm before ordering.

empiric therapy in the meantime. Most labs that perform these tests include an interpretation, but the lab is usually unaware of the patient's presentation and symptoms and may therefore provide an interpretation that is insufficient to guide further management. Slightly abnormal values that are flagged by the lab are not necessarily of clinical significance. In general, communication with a specialist would be prudent to confirm that the results of any advanced test are properly interpreted, even if the result is apparently normal.

ADVANCED METABOLIC SCREENING TESTS

Carnitine

This nutrient is produced by the body and also is available in foods, almost exclusively from animal products (hence the name). Carnitine is essential for the transport of fatty acids into mitochondria where their energy can be released. When the metabolism of fatty acids (and some amino acids) is dysfunctional due to a mutation in a gene in fatty acid breakdown (beta-oxidation), fats become stuck bound to carnitine and both accumulate (causing toxicity) and are wasted (depleting carnitine). Primary carnitine deficiency can be genetic itself. Thus, measuring carnitine is useful for diagnosis and supplementing carnitine can be an important therapy. Patients can also be carnitine deficient due to poor dietary intake (vegan diet), pregnancy, or other chronic conditions and the utility of supplementing carnitine is less clear in these situations.

Plasma acyl-carnitine profile

The acyl-carnitine profile is a catalog of all the fats that are bound to carnitine in the serum. Defects in medium chain acyl-CoA dehydrogenase (the ACADM gene), for example, lead to accumulations of medium chain fats attached to carnitine (predominantly C8, an 8-carbon medium length fat). Many complex patterns of acyl-carnitines can be observed in patients with metabolic conditions, making this a central test in the evaluation of a suspected IEM. This test is also a component of the newborn screen. Very importantly, one must order a free carnitine level separately from the acyl-carnitine profile to assess for carnitine deficiency. An acyl-carnitine profile may not be interpretable if there is a general carnitine deficiency because there may be insufficient carnitine to permit an elevation in any acyl-carnitine species.

Urine organic acids

Organic acids include many familiar compounds, such as lactic acid (lactate) and ketones. Most are more obscure, and are products or intermediates in the metabolism of countless

> **Key Point**
>
> A danger encountered by ICU and emergency medicine physicians is that while labs such as lactate and ammonia return immediately, advanced metabolic studies can take days or even weeks to return results. Lawsuits have resulted from diagnostic metabolic studies that were lost by physicians not accustomed to following labs over long time periods. This concern should encourage systems to follow such labs rather than a hesitancy to send them.

> **Key Point**
>
> Organic acids are best studied in the urine.
> Amino acids are usually studied in the blood.

molecules in the body. Although organic acids are present in the blood, they are substantially concentrated in the urine, making urine the ideal fluid in which to measure them. Urine organic acids are not directly measured on newborn screens and are often helpful in clarifying positive screens.

Plasma amino acids

Many metabolic disorders involve the abnormal metabolism of one or more of the 20 amino acids, as well as several additional amino acids (e.g., ornithine, citrulline) that are not incorporated into polypeptides. Disorders such as phenylketonuria and maple syrup urine disease are detectable by this test. This test is used as part of the newborn screen. After eating, proteins in the meal are hydrolyzed and released directly into the blood from the intestine, and therefore this test is heavily influenced by the most recent meal. A fasting sample is desirable if possible. The duration of appropriate fasting depends on the patient's age. For any unstable patient, testing should be sent immediately. For infants, 2–3 hours after eating is sufficient. For older children, slightly longer is preferable. Obtaining no sample due to a recent meal is less useful than a nonfasting sample. Loading patients with protein in an attempt to exaggerate an abnormal amino acid level should not be attempted.

Orotic acid

This is a precursor in pyrimidine synthesis and in the setting of hyperammonemia an elevated orotic acid suggests the diagnosis of OTC deficiency, a common urea cycle defect because it is X-linked (though girls can be affected, too). This is an important lab to send during any presentation with unexplained hyperammonemia, even in an adult.

Other tests

Countless additional metabolite tests are available. The four listed above (carnitine, acyl-carnitine, organic acids, amino acids) are usually the first-line tests, particularly for a patient in crisis. A specialist may recommend additional tests, emphasizing the need for teamwork when caring for patients with rare IEMs.

SIMPLIFIED APPROACH TO A SUSPECTED INBORN ERROR OF METABOLISM

Many algorithms exist to guide physicians through the differential diagnosis of a suspected IEM based on signs/symptoms and lab values[1] (see Resources). In keeping with the practical goals of this text, we propose a simplified algorithm of broad relevance for any practitioner encountering a patient with a known or suspected IEM:

1. Know the emergency contact information for a metabolic specialist or hospital with metabolic specialists should urgent advice ever be required.

2. Consider that an IEM is on the differential! If the patient has a known diagnosis, he or she should have a letter with a treatment plan, or at least emergency contact information for his or her specialist.

3. Draw essential locally available labs as described above (electrolytes, LFTs, venous blood gas, lactate, ammonia, blood sugar, creatine kinase (CK)).

4. Consider the broader differential and obtain studies (lab, imaging, etc.) as needed.

5. If an IEM is still suspected, speak with a metabolic specialist.

6. Institute a D10+saline infusion at 1.5× maintenance. *Providing abundant carbohydrate calories can be the most important initial management strategy.*

7. If any of the above labs are abnormal, or if an IEM remains a strong diagnostic consideration, send advanced studies:
   a. Acyl-carnitine profile (plasma)
   b. Total and free carnitine (plasma)
   c. Amino acids (plasma)
   d. Organic acids (urine)
   e. Orotic acid (urine, only for unexplained hyperammonemia)
   f. Be prepared to follow these labs until results return

8. Regularly monitor abnormal lab values.

9. Arrange to transfer the patient depending on illness severity and the local availability of critical interventions (e.g., ammonia scavengers, protein-free formula, hemodialysis).

RESOURCES

Pediatrics in Review (http://pedsinreview.aappublications.org/content/30/4/131, http://pedsinreview.aappublications.org/content/30/4/e22)

An overview of inborn errors of metabolism, differential diagnosis, and approach. Pediatrics in Review and the American Association of Pediatrics have other educational resources regarding metabolic disease.

Genetic Metabolic Center for Education (http://www.geneticmetabolic.com)

An organization in the United States committed to making metabolic expertise accessible everywhere given the shortage of specialists in this field. They offer an expanding number of educational options and even clinical consulting.

Urea Cycle Disorders Consortium (https://www.rarediseasesnetwork.org/ucdc/)

An organization dedicated to the study and care of patients with urea cycle disorders. Includes general information as well as treatment guidelines and other resources for urea cycle disorders.

Vademecum Metabolicum[2]

A dense, detailed, and essential handbook of the most known metabolic diseases and their diagnosis and management. Useful to health care practitioners who desire a concise text reference for individual metabolic diseases.

Society for Inherited Metabolic Disorders (http://www.simd.org/links/)

A large organization dedicated to improving education in the field of metabolic disease. Their links section includes links to many other similar societies around the world, labs, and a variety of patient and research groups focused on individual conditions or disease categories.

New England Consortium of Metabolic Programs (http://newenglandconsortium.org/)

A collection of clinical and educational resources for newborn screening, acute illness protocols for metabolic disease, and literature for patients and families.

REFERENCES

1. Burton BK. Inborn errors of metabolism in infancy: a guide to diagnosis. *Pediatrics.* 1998;102(6):E69.
2. Zschocke J, Hoffmann GF. *Vademecum Metabolicum: Diagnosis and Treatment of Inborn Errors of Metabolism.* 3rd ed. Friedrichsdorf: Schattauer; 2011.

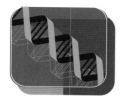

CHAPTER 5

Childhood and Adolescence

The most commonly known genetic disorders diagnosed during childhood and adolescence are developmental delay and autism, although a host of inherited conditions can involve any organ system with onset after the newborn period. Often dubbed "diagnostic dilemmas" because of the difficulty in recognizing them as genetic diseases, these conditions often result in a struggle to establish a diagnosis and effective treatment regimen. Genomic medicine is dramatically impacting genetic disease diagnosis in children, and in some cases leading to life-altering treatment.

AUTISM

A great deal of research in genomics has focused on understanding the genetic pathways that lead to proper or dysfunctional brain development and function. Progress has been made, and much remains to be learned.

As with many childhood genetic diseases, children with autism or developmental delay can be divided into those where the behavioral/cognitive feature is the only symptom, and those that also include other medical problems (e.g., birth defects, dysmorphic/unusual features, abnormal muscle tone). The presence of epilepsy straddles this distinction, as epilepsy is both a component of syndromic causes of autism as well as idiopathic autism. Practitioners who interact with autistic children play a huge role in identifying any other medical concerns, determining the course of intellectual and/or social disability (late onset, regressive, progressive, static), and defining the areas of cognitive function that are impacted (social, spatial, language, etc.).

Role of genetics in autism

A review of the considerable progress in understanding the genetics of autism is beyond the scope of this text. Briefly, twin studies demonstrate that a considerable portion of risk for autism is genetic (possibly >50%), though some environmental contribution must exist. Genetic variation associated with autism currently is understood to consist of[1]:

- Common variants in genes that confer a small risk of autism individually, and must be combined to cause disease. This class of common-but-small-effect variant may contribute relatively less to autism compared to other common disorders (e.g., type II diabetes), or may be too complex in relation to autism to be detected by current techniques. Testing for this type of variant is not yet clinically useful in the diagnosis or management of autism.

- Known genetic syndromes that affect multiple organ systems and include autism, such as Fragile X, tuberous sclerosis, Cowden syndrome, single-gene disorders affecting the Ras pathway (Noonan, Costello, neurofibromatosis type I, cardio-facio-cutaneous syndrome)[2], and others. Identifying this type of cause of autism is particularly important because other health care maintenance may be necessary (e.g., cancer screening).

- Copy number variants CNVs involving deleted or duplicated chromosomal material, usually too small to be detected by karyotype but readily detectable by microarray technology. These may account for approximately 15% of cases of autism and can be diagnosed readily by array technologies[3]. CNVs vary in the quality of the evidence that links them to autism, but several are clearly recognized.

- New (de novo) damaging mutations in a growing list of genes—of which there are likely to be hundreds—that cause autistic features. Some evidence suggests that increased paternal age slightly increases the rate of these spontaneous mutations. Like CNVs, some gene variants are established as causes of autism while others require further evidence.

- Rare variants that are inherited from a parent with variable penetrance for autism. Some evidence indicates that these are more likely to be inherited from the mother, perhaps because autism (for unknown reasons) is less penetrant in females[4]. These, CNVs, and de novo mutations account for most of the recognized genetic contributions to autism.

- Evidence that other types of variation, such as the gut microbiome, epigenetics, and mitochondrial function contribute to autism is only beginning to emerge and time is needed to determine their interaction with better understood pathways and relative contribution to the overall incidence of autism.

Today, by some estimates, 20–40% of children with autism can expect that a plausibly pathogenic genetic variant will be detected either by array or sequencing[5]. Care must be taken in interpreting test results in autistic patients because the quality of the evidence of each gene and each variant within a gene is variable and rapidly changing.

Another important concept in the genetics of autism is that, even in cases where autism appears to be acting like a simple Mendelian disorder, more complexity in terms of inheritance arises than is typical of other conditions. This may be in part due to the fact that autism is more common than typical rare diseases. For example, some children with de novo mutations in known autism genes have autistic siblings who lack this mutation. Family history clearly continues to play a critical role in recurrence risk counseling for families of children with autism[5].

Genetic testing in autism

Guidelines for genetic testing in autism are evolving, but some standards are apparent. In all cases, a careful history and physical must be performed to identify other malformations or involved organ systems that might suggest a unifying syndrome. Evaluation by a child neurologist, developmental pediatrician, psychologist, pediatric psychiatrist, or other professional with expertise in autism is recommended. Routine use of EEG and MRI are probably not indicated in many children with autism who have a normal neurological/ motor exam and no symptoms concerning for seizures, though practices vary and are individualized to each child.

Genetic testing for Fragile X and microdeletion/duplications with a microarray are nearly universal diagnostic practices. Measurement of head circumference often is performed, as mutations in PTEN and CHD8 are associated with both autism and macrocephaly, though familial (benign) macrocephaly is probably more common and unrelated to autism.

Beyond this, approaches vary more widely. Some practitioners undertake metabolic screening (see the section Developmental Delay in this chapter) to identify treatable causes of intellectual disability which can include autistic features, though the yield of such studies is not high if the child had normal newborn screening (though newborn screening is not comprehensive) and lacks other suggestive physical/historical findings (e.g., regression with illness, liver/muscle disease). Numerous vitamin supplements have been suggested to improve autistic symptoms, though unfortunately few if any have stood up to quality clinical trials. Supplementation of branched chain amino acids may partially ameliorate one monogenic cause of autism, but this form is exceedingly rare[6]. Though also rare, creatine synthesis disorders can have autism as a prominent feature and may be treatable with creatine supplementation and a modified diet. Evidence aside, some parents report subjective improvements in behavior with many different dietary manipulations, and within reason such interventions should be supported with appropriate supplementation of missing nutrients such as calcium and vitamin D in dairy-free diets or B12 and/or iron in strictly vegan diets.

Single-gene testing can be performed if the phenotype is typical of a single syndromic form of autism. Autism gene panels that include known (and sometimes merely suspected) autism genes are available from a variety of diagnostics companies (see Appendix 5 for advice on identifying gene panels). These tests offer a compromise between single-gene testing and whole-exome sequencing, with the latter covering more genes at the cost of an increased likelihood of identifying variants that cannot be interpreted. Some specialists perform whole-exome sequencing on all autistic patients, and the field will likely move increasingly in this direction. When ordering exome sequencing for any condition, the practitioner takes on the responsibility of pretest counseling for possible test outcomes as well as thorough variant interpretation (see Appendix 6).

Today, knowledge of the genetic cause of autism leads to a targeted treatment only in a few cases. Nevertheless, knowledge of a causative mutation can help a family understand the diagnosis and allow comparison to other patients with the same affected gene to inform prognosis. Given the limited ability of genetic testing to inform recurrence risk, it remains reasonable for families to defer some testing until technology, cost, and variant interpretation improve. Because autism is an area of highly active research, directing patients and families to trusted studies and trials can both benefit patients as well as advance our understanding of autism.

DEVELOPMENTAL DELAY

Developmental delay possibly is the most common reason for referring a child to a geneticist. Some studies suggest that one-third of patients with developmental delay can be diagnosed by history and physical exam alone, including recognizable syndromes such as Trisomy 21, as well as history suggesting nongenetic causes of delay (e.g., birth asphyxia, trauma, history of meningitis). In other cases, other testing—including genetic testing—may be needed to establish a diagnosis[7-9].

Neuroimaging

Ischemic injuries or brain malformations can cause delay and can be detected by MRI. MRI of the brain indicates an abnormality that explains the delay in about one-third of cases, and more often in patients with focal neurologic exam findings or craniofacial features that frequently co-occur with brain malformations. However, identifying a brain malformation does not necessarily explain *why* the patient has a brain malformation. Both genetic and nongenetic processes (e.g., prenatal infections, stroke, teratogens, or maternal diabetes) can cause brain malformations, and depending on the exact malformation, further study may be needed to provide a more complete diagnosis. That said, uncovering a specific brain malformation can enhance greatly the search for a genetic or other cause of delay and may be of clinical value independent of identifying the underlying etiology. MRI can also show evidence of metabolic disease in the brain based on the location and pattern of abnormal signal. The addition of spectroscopy (sometimes called MRS) if available can aid in the diagnosis of some neurometabolic conditions. Which patients with developmental delay might benefit from neuroimaging is beyond the scope of this text and is best discussed with a child neurologist or other specialist. Geneticists and neurologists—and MRIs and genetic testing—often work hand-in-hand to diagnose children with developmental delay.

Genetic testing: Single-gene tests

Fragile X causes approximately 2% of delay in children. It is difficult to provide an estimate of the diagnostic yield of other single-gene tests because there are thousands of conditions that include developmental delay, the phenotype of each can vary widely and may not be recognizable, and many syndromes can be caused by mutations in more than one gene. In the absence of salient findings on exam and other phenotypic tests, diagnosing a non or mildly dysmorphic child with delay generally requires genome-wide screening approaches.

Chromosomal microarray screening

Chromosomal microarray technology (see Appendix 2) is an established approach (about 10 years old, ancient in terms of genomic techniques though the technology has continued to improve) and currently is the preferred first-line screening tool for children with developmental delay or a host of other potentially genetic conditions unless a particular syndrome is recognized and more targeted testing can be sent. Hundreds of labs offer microarrays. Table 5-1 presents a small sample of commercially available microarrays for postnatal use (they are not intended for prenatal use), in no particular order and with no endorsement of any lab. Microarrays detect submicroscopic (i.e., cannot be seen on a standard karyotype, which is no longer an appropriate first-line screen in most cases) chromosomal deletions or duplications. The diagnostic yield of microarrays is lower in cases of mild delay without other dysmorphic features and increases as the number of involved organ systems increases, with an average yield of approximately 15%.

Metabolic studies

Metabolic disorders can cause developmental delay and are critical to consider because they may be treatable to some extent. Thanks to newborn screening, most children displaying developmental delays will have already had a partial metabolic evaluation as a newborn. In the absence of other signs or symptoms suggestive of a metabolic condition (e.g., regression or waxing/waning neurologic symptoms, involvement of liver or muscle, hyperammonemia/acidosis/hypoglycemia, or certain MRI abnormalities), the diagnostic yield of first-line metabolic screening (acyl-carnitine, amino acid, and organic acid analysis, see Chapter 4) is not high. With the increased application of

Table 5-1. A sample of commercial laboratories offering microarrays for postnatal use.

Laboratory	Test	Link
Quest Diagnostics	ClariSure® Postnatal	http://www.questdiagnostics.com/home/physicians/testing-services/by-test-name/clarisure
ARUP		https://www.aruplab.com/genetics/tests/microarray
Labcorp (via Integrated Genetics)	Reveal SNP Microarray	www.integratedgenetics.com/test-menu/reveal%C2%AE-snp-microarray-pediatric/bbb169c6-2dfc-46ca-aed7-ba13e0efc757
Affymetrix	CytoScan® Dx	http://www.affymetrix.com/estore/browse/staticHtmlContentTemplate.jsp?staticHtmlMediaId=m1861213&isHtmlStatic=true&navMode=35810#1_2

whole-exome sequencing, the number of recognized metabolic disorders has greatly expanded, as has the number of metabolite tests needed to detect each biochemical abnormality. It is important to recognize that many metabolic conditions are not covered by the newborn screen or first-line metabolic screening, such as lysosomal storage diseases, congenital disorders of glycosylation, disorders of creatine metabolism, peroxisomal disorders, disorders of neurotransmitter synthesis, and so on, some of which are treatable. The need for testing with second-line metabolic screens is best considered in consultation with a specialist.

Newer metabolomic technologies that measure hundreds or even thousands of chemicals simultaneously may offer an alternative to sending numerous narrowly focused biochemical tests, but clinical metabolomics currently is too new to assess in any detail. The degree to which exome sequencing and metabolite screening will replace or complement each other remains to be seen, but in general exome sequencing is moving earlier in the diagnostic evaluation.

RARE DISEASES (DIAGNOSTIC DILEMMAS)

There are estimated to be about 8000 rare diseases affecting 30 million (1 in 10) people in the United States, thus collectively diseases are quite common. Most rare diseases affect children and may present as diagnostic dilemmas. Approximately 80% of rare diseases have a genetic basis, and genes for over half of them are currently known (Table 5-2).

Many children with rare genetic diseases become caught in a diagnostic odyssey for years, undergoing countless tests and treatments, emerging with no clear diagnosis and no improvement in their health. According to surveys by the advocacy group Global Genes, it takes an average of 7.6 years for a patient with a rare disease to receive a proper diagnosis in the United States. During this time, patients typically visit up to eight physicians (four primary

Table 5-2. Number of rare genetic diseases by mode of inheritance.

Description	Autosomal	X-linked	Y-linked	Mitochondrial	Total
Molecular basis known	4325	302	4	29	4660
Molecular basis unknown	1503	126	5	0	1634
Additional suspected Mendelian	1694	112	2	0	1808
Total	7522	540	11	29	8102

Data from the Online Mendelian Inheritance in Man (OMIM) database, February 22, 2016

care and four specialists) and receive 2–3 misdiagnoses.[1] These patients are turning increasingly to whole-genome/exome sequencing (WGS/WES) to find the genetic basis of their disease.

Genome and exome sequencing

First available clinically in the United States in 2012, WES has revolutionized the diagnosis of many rare disorders. Both WGS and WES have been employed to uncover the genetic basis of diseases. Given that about 80% of recognized Mendelian disease variants found to date are in the exome, coupled with uncertainty surrounding analysis of nongene-encoding regions found in whole genomes as well as the cost of WGS, WES is more commonly used than WGS at the moment. A growing number of labs offer this test, and most expect that in time WES will merge with microarray testing as a one-size-fits-all screening test for any patient in which a genetic disease is suspected. For the time being it would be most appropriate for this advanced level of testing to be performed with at least some consultation with a specialist, primarily because of the complex results that are returned, the need for pre and posttest counseling, and most importantly the experience needed to be confident that a detected variant is associated with the patient's phenotype.

The broad application of WES to diagnostic dilemmas has already provided several important insights into the science of rare diseases:

- Many classic disorders have wide phenotypic ranges that make atypical cases difficult to diagnose based on clinical features alone. Broad sequencing is necessary.

- Depending on the study, about 5% of patients with complex phenotypes actually have two or more disorders simultaneously, a direct affront to Occam's razor.

- The rate of discovery of new diseases and new gene–phenotype relationships has exploded. It is highly likely that an uncertain variant today will be interpretable in a few years.

Several case series have been published looking at the diagnostic yield of WES in patients with a range of phenotypes and negative workups, and this yield has been consistently approximately 25% (which is impressive when one considers that these patients were not diagnosed by any other means). Importantly, the yield for an individual patient depends on a number of factors:

- Phenotype (most important): Patients with discreet phenotypes involving the eyes, hearing, nervous system, or with multiple congenital anomalies tend to have higher yields (as high as 40–50%), while autism and other less-specific phenotypes have lower yields (about 10–15%). This range reflects many variables, most notably the current state of understanding

---

[1] https://globalgenes.org/wp-content/uploads/2013/04/ShireReport-1.pdf

of the genetic bases of each phenotype. When considering clinical WGS/WES, make sure to provide detailed clinical phenotypes to the testing lab.

- Family history: When multiple family members are affected the likelihood of there being a discreet genetic etiology increases and so does the yield of exome sequencing.
- Trio approach: Sequencing both parents together with the patient allows phase to be determined (if two variants are on the same or different chromosomes) and to identify de novo mutations, a major cause of rare diseases. A recent report found an increased absolute diagnostic yield of about 7% when parents were included[10]. Other affected siblings or family members, when available, can be sequenced as well to improve diagnostic yield.
- Age: Generally, the older the patient (particularly adults), the greater the chance that complex symptoms are acquired rather than genetic. Still, exome sequencing does have an important role to play in adults with suspected genetic diseases[11].
- Timing in overall evaluation: The fewer diseases that have been ruled out before sending exome sequencing, the higher the yield. This does not represent a true characteristic of the exome sequencing itself. Current evidence only reports the yield of WES in patients who have usually had some prior evaluation. Studies are lacking comparing the diagnostic yield of WES in a new patient to a focused evaluation by a specialist. For now, the proper timing of WES in a patient's evaluation is best determined in consultation with a specialist.

Also worth noting is the fact that just as exome sequencing often reveals a diagnosis, some tests reveal a candidate variant that cannot be connected to the phenotype with certainty. Some fraction of these candidate variants are in fact true diagnoses, and the more testing and data collection, the more these variants will be definitively interpretable. Negative exomes can and should be reanalyzed after some time—generally at least 1 year—to determine if new data allows any candidate variants to be reclassified.

Is a patient a candidate for WGS/WES?

A patient on a diagnostic odyssey typically already has undergone extensive clinical evaluation and even focused genetic testing to rule out known genetic diseases. If genetic testing, either single gene or gene panels, for known disorders returns negative results, WGS/WES should be considered[12,13].

How does one select a laboratory for WGS/WES to solve a diagnostic dilemma?

Table 5-3 includes a list of U.S. CLIA-certified laboratories offering clinical diagnostic WGS or WES.

Table 5-3. U.S. CLIA-certified laboratories offering clinical diagnostic whole genome or exome sequencing (in no particular order).

Lab	Website
UCLA Clinical Genomics Center	http://pathology.ucla.edu/body.cfm?id=393
Gene by Gene, Inc.	https://www.genebygene.com/pages/research?goto=exome-sequencing
Laboratory for Molecular Medicine—Harvard Medical School and Partners Healthcare	http://personalizedmedicine.partners.org/Laboratory-For-Molecular-Medicine/Default.aspx
Children's Mercy Hospital and clinics—Molecular Genetics Laboratory	https://www.childrensmercy.org/TestDirectory/testview.aspx?id=2212
Parabase Genomics	http://www.parabasegenomics.com/
GeneDx	https://www.genedx.com/test-catalog/xomedx/
Emory Genetics Laboratory	http://geneticslab.emory.edu/index.html
ARUP Laboratories	http://ltd.aruplab.com/Tests/Pub/2006332
Baylor Miraca Genetics Laboratory	https://www.bcm.edu/research/medical-genetics-labs/test_detail.cfm?testcode=1500
University of Chicago Genetics Services	http://dnatesting.uchicago.edu/tests/670
Cincinnati Children's Hospital Medical Center	https://www.cincinnatichildrens.org/service/d/diagnostic-labs/molecular-genetics/whole-exome-sequencing/
Transgenomic	http://www.transgenomic.com/product/wes-family-specimen-collection-kit/
Medical College of Wisconsin	http://www.mcw.edu/Human-and-Molecular-Genetics-Center-HMGC/Genetic-Diagnostic-Laboratory/Clinical-Sequencing-Services.htm
Personalis	http://www.personalis.com/clinical/
Ambry Genetics Corp	http://www.ambrygen.com/tests/exomenext
Genetics Center	http://www.geneticscenter.com/services/molecular-genetic-laboratory/clinical-exome-sequencing/

Several factors should be considered when selecting a laboratory/test.

Technical considerations:

- *Whole genome versus whole exome*: Over 85% of known mutations for Mendelian diseases occur in the coding region of the genome (exome). Exomes are cheaper and more likely to be covered by insurance. However, whole genomes tend to have more uniform coverage/quality and can detect additional types of variants (large in/dels, translocations, possibly triplet expansions).

- *Coverage/quality*: Minimum average coverage across all sites should be >30× for WES. Lower coverage is needed for WGS. Higher coverage tends to increase cost, but also increases the ability to detect small copy number changes even though WES is not ideally suited to this.

- *Mitochondrial included or not*: Some clinical exomes include the mitochondrial genome while others offer it as an option. The ordering physician must decide if mutations in the mitochondrial genome could plausibly cause the phenotype in question.

- *Microarray analysis*: Currently, most patients for whom exome sequencing is being considered already have had a nondiagnostic microarray. However, as exome sequencing moves earlier in the diagnostic algorithm, one must not forget that current exome technology is not ideal to detect CNVs. Some labs will perform microarrays before or concurrently with exome sequencing if requested.

Services provided:

- *Sequencing only versus sequencing plus diagnostic analysis*: Sequence data alone do not provide a diagnosis. Analysis of sequence data by trained professionals is a key component. Some laboratories only provide the sequence data, while others may outsource sequencing and just do the analysis. Still others may do both. Even the most detailed analyses often require additional literature review to arrive at diagnostic and/or treatment decisions. An ordering physician should know his/her comfort with test interpretation and choose a lab accordingly.

- *Reanalysis*: Data that permits the accurate assignment of uncertain variants as benign or pathogenic are constantly being generated around the world. Some labs actively monitor past whole exome data and provide updates should an important variant be reclassified. Other labs require that a request for reanalysis be formally submitted. Reanalysis of negative exomes after at least about 12 months is highly recommended. Most labs do not charge for the first reanalysis.

- *Return of raw data*: Some laboratories will return the patient's raw sequence data that the ordering physician can then share with others for further analysis or research. Some labs will even share raw data before it is analyzed, while most will not. If this is important, make sure to inquire about the laboratory's data sharing policies.

- *Return of incidental findings*: WGS/WES has the potential to uncover incidental findings in the patient or other family members who have undergone sequence analysis. Some laboratories routinely return these results while others do not. Most have a simple opt-out form, while others allow more complex decisions about what types of incidental findings are desired, if any. This is typically covered during the consenting process.

Practical considerations:

- *Turnaround time*: This ranges from 4 weeks to 24 weeks. Several labs offer expedited exomes available in 1–2 weeks, usually at increased cost and only through institutional billing (i.e., the hospital pays, not the patient's insurance). It is important to consider the urgency of the clinical situation when selecting any genetic test or laboratory.

- *Cost*: WES is cheaper ($1000–9500) than WGS ($7000–18,000). Prices may vary depending on what is included (mitochondrial genome, turnaround time, WES vs. WGS, individual patient vs. family trio, sequencing alone or sequencing plus analysis, etc.). The patient's out of pocket cost also will vary widely, usually based on insurance factors. Importantly, many major labs performing WES/WGS recognize that insurance coverage may be limited and have fee-assistance programs for patients who meet income and other criteria.

- *Insurance coverage/reimbursement*: Probably the greatest obstacle to using diagnostic sequencing is insurance coverage. Countries with single-payer systems have various means to determine if a patient qualifies, for example, for WES, and these standards are applied more or less evenly even though requests may be denied. In the United States, which is a mixture of public and private insurance, coverage varies in the extreme. A myriad of funding sources attempt to fill the gap in coverage, but consistent, evidence-based policies are needed at a higher level. In 2015, Cigna became the first national health plan to articulate a policy on coverage of WGS/WES.[2] WES is covered under their insurance policy for affected individuals meeting specific criteria. Pre and posttest counseling is also covered. WGS is not covered under their policy.

- *Research*: At times, insurance coverage cannot be arranged for WGS/WES and cost is an insurmountable obstacle. Many hospitals and even commercial labs have research protocols that can provide low-cost or free WGS/WES. The downside is that research may come with prolonged

---

[2] https://cignaforhcp.cigna.com/public/content/pdf/coveragePolicies/medical/mm_0519 _coveragepositioncriteria_exome_genome_sequence.pdf

turnaround times (one year or more). The NIH's Rare Diseases Program (https://rarediseases.info.nih.gov/) is one source of information on available research programs.

Pretest counseling and informed consent

It is essential to obtain proper consent and counseling *before* sending WGS/WES testing. Some laboratories have template consent forms on their website and require that it be signed before testing begins. Pretest consent for WGS/WES must address a number of possible results that can come from large scale genomic tests.

- A clear diagnosis.
- No diagnosis with any other findings of potential importance. This can occur if the disorder is not genetic in etiology, if the causative mutation is not detectable by the technology used, or if insufficient data cause an important variant to be overlooked. No lab test is 100% sensitive.
- One or more variants might be found that could be related to the phenotype, but for which adequate data are lacking to confidently associate the variant(s) with the reported phenotype(s). *This is a common outcome.* Further evaluation of these variants may require testing additional family members, deeper investigation into the literature, functional studies when available, and often waiting years for improvement in variant databases.

Several additional unexpected results might occur as well:

- When parents are included in the test, nonpaternity or nonmaternity might be revealed.
- It might be determined that the parents are relatives (consanguinity), if not already recognized.
- A pathogenic variant in a disease-causing gene unrelated to the reason why the test was sent might be uncovered. This could be a cancer risk gene, for example. Patients can opt-out of receiving these results. Importantly, *not* observing such a variant is not proof that it does not exist. *Exome sequencing should not be used as a screen for conditions unrelated to the primary disorder* (e.g., cancer risk, carrier status) unless the ability to do so is explicitly stated by the testing laboratory.
- While the Genetic Information Nondiscrimination Act of 2008 prevents the results of genetic tests from impacting employment and health insurance, it does not prevent their consideration in the issuance of life or disability insurance. How often, if ever, individuals have been affected in terms of life/disability insurance by participating in WGS/WES is not clear.

RARE DISEASES ADVOCACY

It is not uncommon for patients with rare diseases and their families to feel isolated. Several advocacy organizations have been founded to bring together rare disease patients, caregivers, and health care providers. While they might not share the exact same disease, these patients share the same struggles to obtain a diagnosis, access unapproved medicines, finance their journey, etc. Advocacy organizations are an excellent resource for health care providers and patients alike to access the collective wisdom of the rare disease community and useful tools for navigating the rare disease space. Some of the more prominent organizations are listed at the end of the chapter in the Resources section.

At any age, people can present with symptoms that are outside the common diagnoses familiar to most physicians and other providers. The revolution in genomic medicine has made awareness of rare diseases higher than any time in history. Nevertheless, access to this revolution lags behind the technological progress. Everyone plays a role in envisioning a future where individuals with rare diseases have equal access to needed diagnostic and medical care.

RESOURCES

Genetic and Rare Diseases Information Center (GARD) (https://rarediseases .info.nih.gov/gard)

The GARD Information Center was created in 2002 by the Office of Rare Diseases Research (ORDR) and the National Human Genome Research Institute (NHGRI), two agencies of the National Institutes of Health (NIH), to help people find useful information about genetic and rare diseases. The GARD Information Center provides timely access to experienced Information Specialists who provide current and accurate information about genetic and rare diseases in both English and Spanish.

Global Genes (globalgenes.org)

Rare disease advocacy organization building awareness, educating the global community, and providing critical connections and resources that equip advocates to become activists for their disease.

Rare Genomics Institute (http://www.raregenomics.org/)

Provides rare disease patients and families with the necessary tools, knowledge, and connections so that they can better understand the cause of their disease. Brings together scientists, entrepreneurs, innovators, and professionals, and leverages the crowdfunding capabilities of the Internet to bring the hope of a cure to patients. (The ability to crowdfund for genetic testing does not absolve insurers, medical centers, providers, patients, and society from developing better organized means to ensure access to medical care.)

Genetic Alliance (http://www.geneticalliance.org/advocacy)

The most established genetics advocacy group including a network of more than 1200 disease-specific advocacy organizations, as well as thousands of universities, private companies, government agencies, and public policy organizations. The network is an open space for shared resources, creative tools, and innovative programs.

United Mitochondrial Disease Foundation (www.umdf.org)

A large organization that defines mitochondrial disease broadly and seeks to improve research, education, and therapies for these disorders.

SWAN: Syndromes Without A Name (swanusa.org)

A support and advocacy organization for individuals with rare diseases. A similar group in Europe can be found at https://www.undiagnosed.org.uk/

Practice Point: Clinical Scenario

A 3-year-old boy goes to his primary care pediatrician for a well-child checkup. He is behind on his developmental milestones, particularly language and social skills, and his facial features now appear somewhat different from his parents' compared to a year ago. What can the pediatrician do to assist in this child's evaluation?

Points to consider:

1. A careful history is mandatory. When did concerns begin? Has the child lost any skills?
2. A quality physical and neurologic exam are essential. This may include imaging of the abdomen to identify renal anomalies or hepatospleno-megaly, a careful cardiac exam, a skeletal survey to evaluate the bones structurally, and imaging of other parts of the body that may appear affected. Assessment of vision (ideally by an ophthalmologist to assess the structure of the eye and retina) and hearing are also important.
3. Fragile X and chromosomal microdeletion/duplication syndromes (detected by SNP array) are common causes of developmental delay and it is generally reasonable to initiate this evaluation while a referral is pending. It is also reasonable to confer with a specialist before sending these studies.
4. Finally, the child should be referred to a geneticist and/or a child neurologist who is forwarded detailed records of the above findings, with close contact to ensure any other recommended studies are completed. It takes a team to diagnose a rare disease!

REFERENCES

1. De Rubeis S, Buxbaum JD. Genetics and genomics of autism spectrum disorder: embracing complexity. *Hum Mol Genet*. 2015;24(R1):R24-R31. doi:10.1093/hmg/ddv273.
2. Adviento B, Corbin IL, Widjaja F, et al. Autism traits in the RASopathies. *J Med Genet*. 2014;51(1):10-20. doi:10.1136/jmedgenet-2013-101951.
3. Tammimies K, Marshall CR, Walker S, et al. Molecular diagnostic yield of chromosomal microarray analysis and whole-exome sequencing in children with autism spectrum disorder. *JAMA*. 2015;314(9):895-903. doi:10.1001/jama.2015.10078.
4. Iossifov I, Levy D, Allen J, Ye K, et al. Low load for disruptive mutations in autism genes and their biased transmission. *Proc Natl Acad Sci U S A*. 2015;112(41):E5600-5607. doi:10.1073/pnas.1516376112.
5. Geschwind DH, State MW. Gene hunting in autism spectrum disorder: on the path to precision medicine. *Lancet Neurol*. 2015;14(11):1109-1120. doi:10.1016/S1474-4422(15)00044-7.
6. Novarino G, El-Fishawy P, Kayserili H, et al. Mutations in BCKD-kinase lead to a potentially treatable form of autism with epilepsy. *Science*. 2012;338(6105):394-397. doi:10.1126/science.1224631.
7. Sherr EH, Michelson DJ, Shevell MI, Moeschler JB, Gropman AL, Ashwal S. Neurodevelopmental disorders and genetic testing: current approaches and future advances. *Ann Neurol*. 2013;74(2):164-170. doi:10.1002/ana.23950.
8. Flore LA, Milunsky JM. Updates in the genetic evaluation of the child with global developmental delay or intellectual disability. *Semin Pediatr Neurol*. 2012;19(4):173-180. doi:10.1016/j.spen.2012.09.004.
9. Moeschler JB. Genetic evaluation of intellectual disabilities. *Semin Pediatr Neurol*. 2008;15(1):2-9. doi:10.1016/j.spen.2008.01.002.
10. Retterer K, Juusola J, Cho MT, et al. Clinical application of whole-exome sequencing across clinical indications. *Genet Med*. 2015. doi:10.1038/gim.2015.148.
11. Posey JE, Rosenfeld JA, James RA, et al. Molecular diagnostic experience of whole-exome sequencing in adult patients. *Genet Med*. 2015. doi:10.1038/gim.2015.142.
12. Yang Y, Muzny DM, Reid JG, et al. Clinical whole-exome sequencing for the diagnosis of mendelian disorders. *N Engl J Med*. 2013;369(16):1502-1511. doi:10.1056/NEJMoa1306555.
13. de Ligt J, Willemsen MH, van Bon BW, et al. Diagnostic exome sequencing in persons with severe intellectual disability. *N Engl J Med*. 2012;367(20):1921-1929. doi:10.1056/NEJMoa1206524.

ADULTHOOD

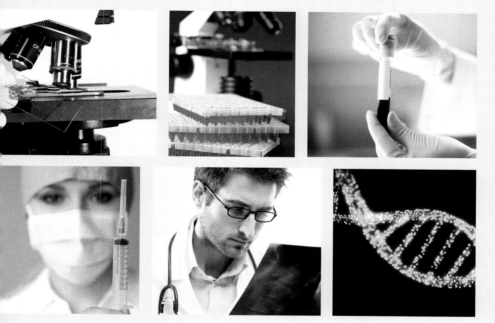

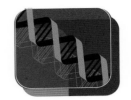

CHAPTER 6

Pharmacogenomics

Pharmaceuticals are prescribed with the assumption that they will provide some benefit to the patient, and will do so safely. Unfortunately, that is not always the case. Commonly used pharmaceuticals are rarely efficacious in everybody. Efficacy varies by drug class, with cancer therapies and Alzheimer's disease drugs on the lower end of the spectrum (Fig. 6-1)[1]. Similarly, pharmaceuticals are not always safe in everybody. Rare and severe adverse events occur in 1–2% of patients (a conservative estimate) and are found across many different therapeutic areas[2].

The application of pharmacogenomics (also called pharmacogenetics) refers to using a patient's genetic information to improve the efficacy and/or reduce the side effects of drugs. Some drugs are only effective in patients with a certain genetic biomarker, in which case a pharmacogenomic test for that biomarker is essential prior to prescribing the drug. This is the case for most of the targeted treatments developed in cancer (reviewed in Chapter 8) and for the cystic fibrosis drugs ivacaftor and lumacaftor/ivacaftor. In other cases the efficacy of a drug may be improved by using a pharmacogenomic test that guides appropriate dosing of the drug. Toxicity-based biomarkers are those that are used to identify people likely to experience side effects when taking the drug. Side effects can range from rare life-threatening adverse events to

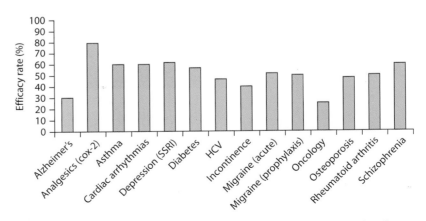

Figure 6-1. **Efficacy of commonly used classes of therapeutics.** (Adapted with permission from Spear BB, Heath-Chiozzi M, Huff J: Clinical application of pharmacogenetics, *Trends Mol Med.* 2001 May;7(5):201-204).

less severe outcomes. Some toxicities can be avoided by either avoiding the drug or adjusting the dose of the drug based on pharmacogenomic tests that reveal the patient's potential to metabolize the drug.

WHEN TO ORDER A PHARMACOGENOMIC TEST

It is estimated that >98% of people in the United States have at least one actionable pharmacogenomic variant from among the 12 most common pharmacogenomic tests, yet most don't know it[3]. That's all changing as several health care institutions (Mayo Clinic, Mt. Sinai Medical Center, St. Judes Children's Research Hospital, University of Florida and Shands Hospital, Vanderbilt University Medical Center) have begun to implement preemptive pharmacogenomic testing programs, making pharmacogenomic information available in the patient medical record prior to any prescribing decision. Preemptive testing will become increasingly common, but until then, when prescribing a drug where there is a known pharmacogenomic association health care providers must decide whether to order a pharmacogenomic test.

There are 138 drugs with pharmacogenomic information in the U.S. Food and Drug Administration (FDA) label (http://www.fda.gov/drugs/scienceresearch/researchareas/pharmacogenetics/ucm083378.htm), the majority (40%) of which are for oncology drugs and discussed in Chapter 8. The clinical validity and utility of the remaining 60% is highly variable. A small number of drugs have pharmacogenomic tests with clear benefit of reducing serious side effects or improving efficacy. These drugs either have language in the FDA label indicating that pharmacogenomic testing is required prior to administration and/or are supported by professional guidelines. Most/all are covered by private insurers or Medicare. These should be on the radar of every health care provider (Table 6-1).

For all other drugs with pharmacogenomic associations, providers should weigh carefully the available evidence supporting the clinical validity of the test, the clinical utility, and the cost/reimbursement, which varies by test and insurance company.

Clinical validity

Clinical validity encompasses how well the pharmacogenomic test can predict the outcome (efficacy/toxicity). Pharmacogenomic tests for rare adverse events tend to have a high negative predictive value, making them useful for ruling out the rare adverse event. For example, among individuals who take allopurinol, a commonly prescribed

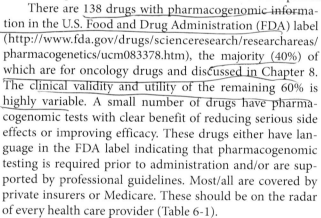

Key Point

Malignant hyperthermia (MH) susceptibility

The operating room is the most common place that a patient first learns that they have susceptibility to MH, a potentially life-threatening reaction to anesthesia (i.e., halothane, isoflurane, sevoflurane, desflurane, and enflurane). MH susceptibility is inherited in an autosomal dominant manner. Mutations in two genes account for most of the cases: *RYR1* (70–80%) and *CACNA1S* (1%). MH is treatable if caught early. According to clinical guidelines, molecular genetic testing is not indicated without likely clinical or biochemical indications of disease, or a family history. However, as genome sequencing becomes more widespread, information about genetic susceptibility to MH should become more readily available and may help patients avoid this serious reaction to anesthesia. For more information, see GeneReviews (http://www.ncbi.nlm.nih.gov/books/NBK1146/).

Table 6-1. Pharmacogenomic tests with a very strong evidence base.

Therapeutic area	Drug	Gene/Variant	PharmGKB drug label interpretation	Guidelines	Use
Cystic fibrosis	Kalydeco® (ivacaftor)	CFTR/G551D and others	Required	CPIC	Efficacy
Cystic fibrosis	Orkambi™ (lumacaftor/ ivacaftor)	CFTR/F508Del	—		Efficacy
HIV/AIDS	Ziagen® (abacavir)	HLA-B*5701	Recommend	CPIC, DHHS	Avoid toxicity
Epilepsy	Tegretol® (carbamazepine)	HLA-B*1502	Required	CPIC, CPNDS	Avoid toxicity
Epilepsy	Tegretol® (carbamazepine)	HLA-A*31:01		CPNDS	Avoid toxicity
Gout	Krystexxa® (pegloticase)	G6PD deficiency	Required (EMA)	EPAR	Avoid toxicity
Tourette's	ORAP® (pimozide)	CYP2D6 PM	Required	—	Avoid toxicity
Huntington's	Xenazine® (tetrabenazine)	CYP2D6 PM	Required	—	Avoid toxicity

This list was compiled by reviewing tests in the CDC tier 1 classification (www.cdc.gov/genomics/gtesting/tier.htm) and PharmGKB Level 1 required classification (www .pharmgkb.org/view/drug-labels.do) of pharmacogenomic tests. CPIC, Clinical Pharmacogenomics Implementation Consortium; ACR, American College of Rheumatology; DHHS, Department of Health and Human Services; CPNDS, Canadian Pharmacogenomics Network for Drug Safety; EPAR, European Public Assessment Report; EMA, European Medicines Agency; PM, poor metabolizer.

medication for gout and hyperuricemia, about 4/1000 will experience severe cutaneous adverse reactions (SCAR), which include the drug hypersensitivity syndrome, Stevens–Johnson syndrome, and toxic epidermal necrolysis. Nearly all of the patients with SCAR will have HLA-B*5801, a variant found in 20% of the general population. Therefore, this variant is necessary, but not sufficient for developing SCAR and individuals who test negative for HLA-B*5801 can safely take the drug. The positive predictive value, or risk of SCAR in someone who has the HLA-B*5801 is low, only about 2.6%, not that much greater than the risk of SCAR in general (0.4%). However, because of the seriousness of the side effect, even this small increased risk may be too great for patients to assume, especially if an alternative treatment is available.

Clinical utility

Clinical utility of pharmacogenomic tests refers to whether the test will impact health care decisions and have a favorable risk/benefit profile. Health care decisions associated with pharmacogenomic test results include adjusting the dose of the drug, increased monitoring, or avoiding the drug altogether and instead, considering alternative treatments if available.

Clinical utility is also dependent on the risk/benefit of deviating from the recommended drug dose. For example, patients who test positive for a pharmacogenomic test for irinotecan-associated neutropenia should receive a lower dose to avoid neutropenia. However, this test was not recommended in a systematic review by the Evaluation of Genomic Applications in Practice and Prevention Working Group because the risk to the patient of developing neutropenia was deemed less than the risk of inefficacy against the cancer because the patient received a subtherapeutic dose[4].

Randomized controlled clinical trials are the gold standard for demonstrating clinical utility, but this bar may be unrealistic to reach for rare adverse events or pharmacogenomic markers relevant to a subset of patients with an already uncommon disease (e.g., cancer patients with specific tumor markers). Unlike many other genetic tests, pharmacogenomic tests have clearer utility in terms of affecting treatment decisions, but whether those decisions lead to improved outcomes or reduced health care costs is not always clear. When deciding on whether to use a pharmacogenomic test or not, practitioners should consider how important having clearly demonstrated clinical utility is to them and their patient.

A few additional points to make about when to order a test:

- Pharmacogenomic testing may have a larger impact on drugs that have a narrow therapeutic window than those with a wide one. For example, the anticoagulant warfarin, used to prevent thromboembolism, puts patients at risk of hemorrhage at higher doses. Both safety and efficacy are paramount and dependent on adequate but not excessive dosing of the drug, which in this case lies in a narrow range.

- Many drugs are already prescribed in a way that maximizes safety and minimizes the risk of side effects by starting at a low dose and increasing dose as tolerated. Simply relying on blood biochemistry to monitor response to the drug, as is done with the international normalized ratio (INR) for warfarin, and adjusting drug levels accordingly, may be sufficient.

- Some pharmacogenomic tests are relevant to specific drugs in a class, while others are relevant to the entire class. For example, simvastatin-associated myopathy is linked to variation in the *SLCO1B1* gene, but other statins like atorvastatin are less dependent on this variation and may be prescribed instead of simvastatin in patients with increased risk of myopathy[5]. In contrast, because tricyclic antidepressants have similar pharmacokinetic properties, dosing guidelines based on variation in *CYP2D6* and *CYP2C19* may be applicable to all drugs in that class.

Summary of questions to ask when considering a pharmacogenomic test:

- Are there alternative drugs that could be used that would not require pharmacogenomic testing?
- If the patient tests positive for a marker associated with an increased relative risk of toxicity, what would be the absolute risk of an adverse event? Would it be worth using a different drug?
- Are other (possibly less expensive or more accessible) means of monitoring for toxicity available?

WHERE TO FIND INFORMATION ABOUT SPECIFIC PHARMACOGENOMIC TESTS

Information about the pharmacogenomic tests can be obtained from various sources including the drug label, evidence guidelines, and the PharmGKB website.

The drug label

The first place one might learn about a pharmacogenomic biomarker is from the drug label. In 2006, the U.S. FDA began to include pharmacogenomic data into existing drug labels, based on recommendations from an expert advisory committee. Twelve percent of the 385 drugs approved by the FDA between 1998 and 2012 have pharmacogenomic biomarker data in their label. There are a few important things to know about pharmacogenomic information and drug labels:

- Some drugs with pharmacogenomic tests do not currently contain this information in the drug label (e.g., simvastatin and *SLCO1B1*, allopurinol and *HLA-B*), despite the associations having been known for years.
- The drug label does not typically address the clinical validity of the pharmacogenomic test. Just because information about a pharmacogenomic marker is included in the drug label, don't assume that the test has clinical validity, much less clinical utility.
- The placement of pharmacogenomic information in the label is not standardized. It can appear in any section of the label and often in multiple sections. Moreover, the location does not seem to correlate well with the importance of the test, in terms of how necessary it is for avoiding toxicity or ensuring efficacy. For example, the Boxed Warning section for clopidogrel contains information about pharmacogenomic testing, but the validity and importance of this test is controversial.
- The vocabulary used to describe pharmacogenomic information in a drug label is not standardized, leading to confusion about the importance of the pharmacogenomic biomarker. For example, "It is recommended

that consideration be given to either genotype or phenotype patients for TPMT" in the label for Azathioprine and Individuals who are homozygous for the *UGT1A1*28* allele are at increased risk for neutropenia following treatment in the label for Irinotecan. Neither description speaks of the importance of testing.

Evidence guidelines

Evidence guidelines for the use of pharmacogenomic testing come from various professional organizations and usually include recommendations on whether a test should be ordered or not, but these guidelines are sparse. Guidelines can be searched for at the National Guidelines Clearinghouse (www.guideline.gov/). Another excellent resource for locating a summary of available guidelines for pharmacogenomics can be found at the Community Pharmacist Pharmacogenetics Network (rxpgx.com/).

The Clinical Pharmacogenomics Implementation Consortium (CPIC) is an organization that produces pharmacogenomic guidelines that assume testing has already occurred and results are already available, as in the case of preemptive testing. They do not suggest whether a test should be ordered or not, but rather, how to interpret test results and make treatment decisions when test results are already available.

Other organizations producing pharmacogenomic guidelines include: the Dutch Pharmacogenomics Working Group; the Canadian Pharmacogenomics Network for Drug Safety; and the European Medicines Agency.

PharmGKB

PharmGKB (www.pharmgkb.org) is one of the most comprehensive public resources for implementing pharmacogenomics. It integrates information from the drug label and evidence guidelines into a searchable knowledgebase. PharmGKB curates and grades the evidence supporting pharmacogenomic tests and provides dosing recommendations based on CPIC guidelines through a simple web-based interface.

UNDERSTANDING THE CYTOCHROME P450 GENES

Among the pharmacogenomic markers in drug labels, a few stand out as being relevant to multiple drugs. These include three genes in the cytochrome P450 (CYP) family, *CYP2D6*, *CYP2C19*, and *CYP2C9*, which encode enzymes responsible for metabolism of endogenous and exogenous compounds, including pharmaceuticals. Some drugs, like the anticoagulant warfarin, are active compounds that are metabolized by CYP enzymes (in this case *CYP2C9*) into inactive compounds prior to excretion. For other drugs, CYP enzymes are responsible for activating the drug, as is the case with the prodrug codeine, which is metabolized by *CYP2D6* into the active compound, morphine. An estimated three-quarters of therapeutic agents are metabolized by one or more of these enzymes. There is large interindividual variation in the activity of the CYP enzymes. Most people have normal functioning enzymes and are considered *extensive metabolizers* (EM). Others have reduced functioning enzymes and are considered either *intermediate metabolizers* (IM) or *poor metabolizers* (PM). Still other individuals have enzymes that appear to be overactive and are considered *ultrarapid metabolizers* (UM).

This profound interindividual variation in enzyme activity is based in large part on underlying genetic variation in the CYP genes. For example, gene duplication events can lead to a person inheriting an extra copy of a CYP gene, resulting in a phenotype of UM. IMs and PMs typically have whole gene deletions, variable sized insertion/deletions, or point mutations that impact enzyme structure and function. In addition, all individuals will also have some gene variants that are silent and have no effect on the enzyme activity.

Certain combinations of variants appear together frequently in the gene and for simplicity's sake, these *alleles* are named using a star and number (e.g., *1, *2, *3, etc.). Dozens of alleles have been described for the various CYP genes, including 35 for *CYP2C19*, 60 for *CYP2C9*, and 105 for *CYP2D6*. Each allele is associated with an enzyme activity (increased, decreased), and each pair of alleles in a person can be related to the metabolizer phenotypes (PM, EM, IM, UM). The Karolinska Institute hosts a CYP nomenclature website that tracks and defines the genetic composition of alleles discovered to date, as well as the corresponding enzyme activity (www.cypalleles.ki.se).

A typical CYP will have 2–4 alleles that are relatively common in the population and then a long tail of rare alleles that affect only a small proportion of individuals (Fig. 6-2). There are likely to be even more novel alleles that will be discovered as more individuals have their CYP genes sequenced. CYP allele frequencies vary by ethnicity, with some being more common in one ethnic group compared to another.

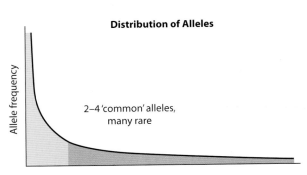

Distribution of Alleles

Allele frequency

2–4 'common' alleles,
many rare

Figure 6-2. **A typical CYP will have 2-4 alleles that are relatively common in the population and then a long tail of rare alleles that affect only a small proportion of individuals.**

LABORATORY TESTS FOR PHARMACOGENOMIC MARKERS

The most comprehensive method for detecting all possible variation in pharmacogenes, including both known and novel variants, is gene sequencing. The drawbacks of sequencing include cost and interpretation: the effect of any newly discovered variants on the function of the downstream protein will require further investigation that is generally not available as a clinical test. Instead, most laboratories will carry out multiplex *targeted* genotyping of known alleles, which is probably sufficient. Sometimes different complementary methodologies are required to test for simple single nucleotide changes versus gene duplications and deletions.

Laboratories usually perform targeted genotyping on only a subset of all known alleles in a given pharmacogene, typically the most common ones. For example a survey of 14 laboratories conducting *CYP2C19* testing found that, although at least seven alleles leading to poor metabolism are known, most labs only test for the two most common ones (*2 and *3)[6]. Similarly, there is a common well-known allele, *CYP2C19*17, leading to ultrarapid drug metabolism, but only 60% of labs tested for it. Pratt et al[7] published an excellent review of different testing assays used by laboratories for the most common CYP genes and their performance on a reference panel of cell lines.

The result of only testing for a subset of all known alleles is possible misclassification, which impacts the test's analytical validity. For example platforms that don't detect the *CYP2D6*41 allele, a known reduced function allele,

---

Practice Point: Clinical Scenario

A surgical patient reveals during their preop visit that the last time they had oral surgery and received codeine for pain, they fainted and are now apprehensive about taking codeine. Do you offer them pharmacogenomic testing before administering or prescribing any codeine prior to surgery?

Consider the following:

1. Is there a clinically valid pharmacogenomic test available for codeine that may inform your decision? To find out, review the PharmGKB website.
2. Is there an alternate treatment available? If so, you may just choose to use the alternate drug and forego testing. (In fact, the use of codeine is discouraged in all children independent of pharmacogenetic testing because of the risk of side effects.)
3. If dosing adjustments are suggested, does the potential benefit of possible under or overdosing to reduce side effects outweigh the risk of the drug not effectively managing pain?

may misclassify the person as having *CYP2D6*2* instead, which is a normal functioning allele. Laboratories may differ in their interpretation of variants as well. A person with one copy of the *CYP2C19*17* allele is typically classified as an ultrarapid metabolizer, but 29% of laboratories classified these cases as normal metabolism in the same study[7]. A practitioner may need to know what precise alleles are important for the drug in question to choose a test.

Several laboratories offer pharmacogenomic testing. To find a laboratory and test, visit the NIH Genetic Testing Registry (http://www.ncbi.nlm.nih.gov/gtr/), NextGxDx (www.nextgxdx.com), or other sites described in Appendix 5.

FUTURE CHALLENGES AND OPPORTUNITIES IN PHARMACOGENOMICS

The biggest challenge facing pharmacogenomics is the lack of sufficient evidence in support of clinical validity and utility of the tests. This evidence drives coverage decisions and ultimate uptake by health care providers. In the absence of clear and consistent evidence, the burden falls on the health care provider to evaluate the potential benefit and risk of pharmacogenomic testing. Resources like PharmGKB are invaluable for this purpose, but require time and effort to access and review.

Efficient deployment of pharmacogenomics will require integration into the flow of medical practice. Several groups are working on clinical decision support to facilitate ordering of pharmacogenomic tests[8-10]. Others have piloted preemptive pharmacogenomic testing and developed infrastructure to store that information in the electronic health record[11, 12]. As genome sequencing becomes a routine part of health care, technological challenges related to collecting genomic data will eventually be overcome, though the accumulation of quality outcomes data will require a longer term process. Until then, health care providers should familiarize themselves with the most common use cases for pharmacogenomics and the resources available for evaluating and implementing these tests into practice.

RESOURCES

PharmGKB (www.pharmgkb.org)

The PharmGKB is a pharmacogenomics knowledge resource that encompasses clinical information including dosing guidelines and drug labels, potentially clinically actionable gene–drug associations and genotype–phenotype relationships. PharmGKB collects, curates, and disseminates knowledge about the impact of human genetic variation on drug responses.

Community Pharmacist Pharmacogenetics Network (rxpgx.com)

The CPPN aims to provide community pharmacists with the resources they need to deliver pharmacogenetic testing efficiently and effectively, including links to guidelines, patient materials, laboratories, and a blog.

SNPits (http://personalizedmedicine.ufhealth.org/snp-its/pharmacogenomics
-study-summaries/)

SNP•its from the University of Florida produces study summaries and inter-pretations of clinical pharmacogenomics research written by clinical phar-macists for other pharmacists, health care professionals, and researchers. They use an evidence-based approach to answer questions about the impli-cations of pharmacogenomics research for patient care: What do clinical guidelines say about a specific drug–gene pair reviewed in a recent study? What is the quality of the evidence supporting genotype-guided therapy? How are pharmacogenomic test results interpreted to guide drug therapy changes?

Table of pharmacogenomic markers on drug labels (www.fda.gov/drugs/
scienceresearch/researchareas/pharmacogenetics/ucm083378.htm)

List maintained by the U.S. Food and Drug Administration of all FDA-approved drugs with pharmacogenomic information in the label, the phar-macogenomic marker, and the location of the pharmacogenomic information in the drug label.

Clinical Pharmacogenomics Implementation Consortium (www.pharmgkb
.org/page/cpic)

Consortium that develops guidelines designed to help clinicians understand how available genetic test results should be used to optimize drug therapy, rather than *whether* tests should be ordered.

Dutch Pharmacogenomics Working Group (DPWG) (https://www.pharmgkb
.org/page/dpwg)

A multidisciplinary organization established in 2005 by the Royal Dutch Pharmacist's Association with the objectives of developing pharmaco-genetics-based therapeutic (dose) recommendations and assisting drug prescribers and pharmacists by integrating the recommendations into computerized systems for drug prescription and automated medication surveillance.

CDC Office of Public Health Genomics (OPHG) classification of genetic tests (www.cdc.gov/genomics/gtesting/tier.htm)

Results of horizon scanning to identify and track the progress of genomic tests as they move from research into clinical and public health practice. As an aid in organizing horizon scanning results, OPHG ranks genomic tests, and family health history applications, by levels of evidence.

REFERENCES

1. Spear BB, Heath-Chiozzi M, Huff J. Clinical application of pharmacogenetics. *Trends Mol Med.* 2001;7:201-204.
2. Hakkarainen KM, Hedna K, Petzold M, Hagg S. Percentage of patients with preventable adverse drug reactions and preventability of adverse drug reactions—a meta-analysis. *PLoS One.* 2012;7:e33236.

3. Dunnenberger HM, Crews KR, Hoffman JM, et al. Preemptive clinical pharmacogenetics implementation: current programs in five US medical centers. *Annu Rev Pharmacol Toxicol.* 2015;55:89-106.
4. Evaluation of Genomic Applications in Practice and Prevention (EGAPP) Working Group. Recommendations from the EGAPP Working Group: can UGT1A1 genotyping reduce morbidity and mortality in patients with metastatic colorectal cancer treated with irinotecan? *Genet Med.* 2009;11:15-20.
5. Canestaro WJ, Austin MA, Thummel KE. Genetic factors affecting statin concentrations and subsequent myopathy: a HuGENet systematic review. *Genet Med.* 2014;16:810-819.
6. van Schaik R. Clinical application of pharmacogenetics: where are we now? *J Int Fed Clin Chem Lab Med.* 2013;24:1-8.
7. Pratt VM, Zehnbauer B, Wilson JA, et al. Characterization of 107 genomic DNA reference materials for CYP2D6, CYP2C19, CYP2C9, VKORC1, and UGT1A1: a GeT-RM and Association for Molecular Pathology collaborative project. *J Mol Diagn.* 2010;12:835-846.
8. Bell GC, Crews KR, Wilkinson MR, et al. Development and use of active clinical decision support for preemptive pharmacogenomics. *J Am Med Inform Assoc.* 2014;21:e93-e99.
9. Devine EB, Lee CJ, Overby CL, et al. Usability evaluation of pharmacogenomics clinical decision support aids and clinical knowledge resources in a computerized provider order entry system: a mixed methods approach. *Int J Med Inform.* 2014;83:473-483.
10. Nishimura AA, Shirts BH, Dorschner MO, et al. Development of clinical decision support alerts for pharmacogenomic incidental findings from exome sequencing. *Genet Med.* 2015;17:939-942.
11. Rasmussen-Torvik LJ, Stallings SC, Gordon AS, et al. Design and anticipated outcomes of the eMERGE-PGx project: a multicenter pilot for preemptive pharmacogenomics in electronic health record systems. *Clin Pharmacol Ther.* 2014;96:482-489.
12. Bielinski SJ, Olson JE, Pathak J, et al. Preemptive genotyping for personalized medicine: design of the right drug, right dose, right time-using genomic data to individualize treatment protocol. *Mayo Clin Proc.* 2014;89:25-33.

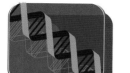

CHAPTER 7

Heart Disease

Precision medicine is being applied in several areas of cardiovascular disease. Various tests are available to identify individuals with hereditary predisposition to familial hypercholesterolemia, inherited thrombophilia, arrhythmias, cardiomyopathy, and other rare genetic heart defects. Pharmacogenomic tests are being considered for commonly prescribed drugs including clopidogrel, warfarin, and simvastatin. What are the indications for these tests? Are they clinically valid and useful? Where can you learn more?

CORONARY ARTERY DISEASE

Coronary artery disease, the most common manifestation of cardiovascular disease, has long been suspected to have an inherited component, especially when it occurs prematurely. However, despite best efforts in the field of genomics to identify high-risk genetic variants underlying the disease, few such variants exist. Most genetic variants for coronary artery disease discovered to date are common variants with very small effects (low-risk variants).

Common variants

Common genetic variants in over 33 gene regions, including the *APOE* gene and the genomic region 9p21, have been reproducibly shown to be associated with coronary artery disease risk (Table 7-1). Most (70%) of these genetic variant associations are independent of known risk factors[1]. The average magnitude of increased risk associated with each variant is very small, on average 1.18-fold. For example, if the average population risk of coronary artery disease is 25%, carriers of one of these low-risk variants would be at about 29.5% risk. Clinical validity of these common low-risk genetic variants has not been demonstrated and no current guidelines support genetic testing[2]. Researchers have tried to develop aggregate risk prediction scores from multiple common low-risk variants, but none of these have yet been validated in prospective studies[3].

Familial hypercholesterolemia (FH)

FH is one exception of a genetic risk factor for coronary artery disease, where rare variants in one of three genes, *LDLR, APOB,* and *PCSK9*, are associated in an autosomal dominant fashion with severely elevated low-density lipoprotein (LDL) cholesterol levels and high risk of premature

Table 7-1. Characteristics of common genetic variants associated with risk of coronary artery disease.

Gene/region	Risk variant	Variant frequency	Relative risk of CAD	Risk (penetrance) of CAD in carriers
9p21	Rs10757278	75%	1.2–1.4	30–35%[a]
APOE	E4 (rs7412 and rs429358)	25%	1.06	26.5%[a]
LDLR	Many	<1%	3.6[b]	Up to 90%
APOB	Many	<1%		Unknown
PCSK9	Many	<1%	3.6[b]	Up to 90%

CAD, coronary artery disease.
[a] Estimated assuming general population risk of 25%; risks from genome-wide association studies.
[b] Derived from penetrance estimates cited in GeneReviews and assuming general population risk of 25%.

myocardial infarction. FH is common, affecting approximately 1:200 to 1:500 people, but the prevalence varies by population[4]. FH is treatable, with lipid-lowering therapy increasing survival and decreasing morbidity[5]. Clinical management guidelines and other useful information about FH are summarized in GeneReviews (http://www.ncbi.nlm.nih.gov/books/NBK174884/).

Although guidelines from the National Lipid Association suggest that genetic testing is not typically needed for a diagnosis, it is useful when laboratory results are uncertain (NLA lipid.org). Uncertainty becomes more common at older ages where cholesterol levels increase naturally and there is overlap between FH and non-FH[6]. Identification of causal mutations may provide motivation for patients to adhere to treatment. European studies also suggest that cascade screening efforts (family tracing) can be improved by algorithms that include genetic testing.

Genetic testing for FH is one of only three genetic tests classified as a Tier 1 test by the Office of Public Health Genomics of the U.S. Centers for Disease Control and Prevention, indicating a test with established clinical utility.[1] Unlike the *APOE* gene and 9p21 gene region for coronary artery disease, where a single common risk variant has been identified, FH is characterized by allelic heterogeneity. In other words, hundreds of rare, high-risk pathogenic mutations have been identified in each of the three genes (Table 7-1). Many laboratories offer testing for FH, but some only test for the most common causes of FH, mutations in the *LDLR* gene (accounting for 60–80% of cases). Mutations in two other genes also contribute to the

[1] http://www.cdc.gov/genomics/gtesting/tier.htm

burden of FH, including *APOB* (1–5%) and *PCSK9* (1–3%), and should be considered as well.

HEREDITARY THROMBOPHILIAS

Hereditary thrombophilia is associated with common genetic variants in several genes, including those encoding factor V Leiden, prothrombin, antithrombin III, protein C, and protein S. The factor V Leiden variant accounts for the greatest proportion, found in 15–20% of individuals with a first deep vein thrombosis. This variant is most common in individuals with European ancestry, and least common in Asians. Heterozygosity for the prothrombin variant (20210G>A in the *F2* gene) is also present in a few percent of Europeans (Table 7-2). The other risk variants are less common but also recognized to increase the risk of thrombosis. Genetic tests for inherited thrombophilias are targeted genotyping tests. In other words, the specific variants, factor V Leiden and prothrombin 20210G>A, are the only relevant variants and can easily be genotyped with a number of different genotyping platforms.

The common variants in *MTHFR* (C677T and A1298C) are not mentioned here because evidence that these variants cause any health effects is conflicting and generally poor. In fact, in the Choosing Wisely® program, the American College of Medical Genetics and Genomics (ACMG) recommends against testing this gene as part of an evaluation for hereditary thrombophilia. The American College of Obstetrics and Gynecology (ACOG) similarly questions the value of testing this gene for women's health.

Table 7-2. Genetic factors commonly associated with venous thromboembolism.

Gene	*F2* (Factor II)	*F5* (Factor V)
Variant	20210G>A; RS1799963	Leiden (Arg506Gln; 1691G>A; RS6025)
Relative risk for one copy[7]	3	5
Relative risk for 2 copies[7]	Not well defined	10
U.S. European frequency[8],a	2–5%	5.2%
U.S. Hispanic frequency	2.2%	2.2%
U.S. African frequency	<1%	1.2%
U.S. Asian/Native Am frequency	<1%	<1%
Gene Reviews	/NBK1148/	/NBK1368/

a http://www.cdc.gov/ncbddd/dvt/data.html

Screening for hereditary thrombophilia

Broad screening

At first glance, it would seem obvious that screening for risk-conferring variants of thrombophilia genes, especially factor V and prothrombin, would be important for everyone, but broad screening is rarely so simple, for the following reasons:

- Especially for younger individuals, the absolute risk of thrombosis is low (1–2 per 1000 per year in the United States) and remains low even in variant carriers.

- Anticoagulant medications such as warfarin and heparin used for treatment to prevent thrombosis are not without risks, and anticoagulating a healthy individual for a lifetime would be a major intervention.

- Those with a personal and/or family history of thrombosis may already be candidates for increased surveillance or anticoagulation during high-risk situations, and medical and family histories are rapid and free to obtain.

Screening in pregnancy and birth control

Perhaps the most common situations where thrombophilia risk may be clinically actionable are when considering birth control options and during pregnancy. ACOG has issued a practice guideline on this topic that covers various risk genes and alleles, testing recommendations, and anticoagulation regimens based on genetics, and is worth reviewing for those who practice in this field.[2] It is important to note that these guidelines vary in the degree of clinical evidence available to support them.

What is important to note from these guidelines is that while in some situations anticoagulation during pregnancy may be recommended based on genotype alone, it is not recommended that women be universally screened. For this reason, it is inevitable that a high-risk woman won't receive anticoagulation because she wasn't screened, but she will most likely suffer no ill effects. For example, per the ACOG guidelines,[3] a factor V Leiden homozygous woman with no history of thrombosis would only have a 4% chance of having a venous thromboembolism during a pregnancy.

With regard to birth control, many gynecologists will not prescribe estrogen-containing contraceptives to a woman known to have a genetic risk factor for thrombosis. However, pregnancy confers an even higher risk of thrombosis, and thus effective contraception (when desired) should not be compromised due to a genetic risk alone.

---

[2] ACOG Practice Bulletin Number 138, September 2013.

[3] ACOG Practice Bulletin Number 138, September 2013.

RARE MONOGENIC HEART DEFECTS

Inherited cardiac defects are a major cause of premature and sudden cardiac death (SCD). Screening for pathogenic variants underlying cardiomyopathies (e.g., hypertrophic cardiomyopathy (HCM) and cardiac channelopathies (Long QT syndrome, LQTS)), both known causes of SCD, has become standard of care and can inform risk to family members of affected individuals and in some cases allow presymptomatic treatment. Postmortem genetic testing (molecular autopsies) in the case of SCD can provide closure to family members, as well as inform risk to family members.

In general, genetic testing may be more informative in persons with clinical disease, where the prior probability of a rare disease-causing variant is higher compared to healthy individuals (see Appendix 6 regarding interpretation of variants). As a case in point, a study of genetic testing of two well-known arrhythmia genes in an unselected cohort of subjects without previously known arrhythmias found that subjects with putative pathogenic variants were no more likely to have evidence of arrhythmia in their medical records than those without pathogenic variants[9].

Results of genetic testing are useful for understanding lifestyle triggers in some cases; for example, different genetic subtypes of LQTS are triggered by exercise, sleep, or emotional stimuli. Individuals with an inherited predisposition may be advised to alter lifestyle, increase surveillance, initiate prophylactic medication, or consider an implantable cardioverter-defibrillator. The invasiveness of some of these interventions also highlights the importance of avoiding unnecessary testing and uninterpretable results. Once a causal mutation is identified in an affected individual, it may prompt genetic testing of that very same variant and/or clinical screening for signs of disease in other unaffected family members. Table 7-3 lists rare monogenic heart conditions where genetic tests are available. Clinical management guidelines can be found at GeneReviews (http://www.ncbi.nlm.nih.gov/books/NBK1116/).

Guidelines

The European Heart Rhythm Association and the Heart Rhythm Society addresses a wide range of genetic heart diseases in their guidelines and recommend the following[10]:

1. Genetic testing for LQTS, catecholaminergic polymorphic ventricular tachycardia (CPVT), dilated cardiomyopathy (DCM), and HCM in patients with a clinical suspicion of the disorder. (Note: There are several nuances among the criteria for testing. Other disorders are mentioned, but testing is not recommended, rather, it states that testing "can be useful" or may be considered for other disorders including Brugada syndrome (BrS), progressive cardiac conduction disease (CDD), short QT syndrome (SQTS), arrhythmogenic cardiomyopathy (ACM)/arrhythmogenic right

Table 7-3. Available genetic tests for rare monogenic heart defects.

Phenotype/disease	Gene Reviews
Arrhythmias	
Long QT syndrome	
Romano-Ward syndrome	NBK1129/
Jervell–Lange-Nielsen syndrome	NBK1405/
Andersen–Tawil syndrome	NBK1264/
Timothy syndrome	NBK1403/
Brugada syndrome	NBK1517/
Cardiomyopathies	
Hypertrophic cardiomyopathy	NBK1768/
Dilated cardiomyopathy	NBK1309/
Arrhythmogenic right ventricular cardiomyopathy/dysplasia	NBK1131/
Marfan, aneurysm, and aortopathies	
Marfan syndrome	NBK1335/
Ehlers–Danlos syndrome type IV	NBK1494/
Loeys–Dietz syndrome	NBK1133/
Familial thoracic aortic aneurysm and dissection	NBK1120/

ventricular cardiomyopathy (ARVC), left ventricular noncompaction (LVNC), and restrictive cardiomyopathy (RCM).)

2. Targeted genetic testing of family members of patients in whom a causative mutation is found is recommended for all of these genetic heart diseases.

3. Postmortem genetic testing for genetic heart diseases in cases of sudden unexplained death or sudden infant death syndrome.

The American College of Cardiology Foundation and The American Heart Association recommend the following[4]:

1. Genetic testing for HCM and other genetic causes of unexplained cardiac hypertrophy in patients with an atypical clinical presentation or when another genetic condition is suspected.

2. Screening (either clinical or with genetic testing) in first-degree relatives of patients with HCM.

3. Genetic counseling and assessment of family history as part of evaluation of HCM.

Choosing a laboratory and test

Dozens of laboratories offer tests for monogenic heart defects, ranging from single-gene tests to larger gene panels to comprehensive exome sequencing. The number of genes tested for a given condition can vary widely between laboratories. A more in-depth discussion about how to find a lab, choose and order an appropriate gene panel, and interpret results can be found in Appendices 5 and 6, respectively. In general, it is a good idea to read the GeneReviews summary to understand what the most important genes are to test. A variety of options are available for testing narrowly defined phenotypes (e.g., a two-gene panel for Jervell–Lange-Nielsen syndrome) versus a broader phenotype (e.g., 30–60 gene arrhythmia panels). These conditions are typically inherited in either a dominant or recessive fashion and are characterized by genetic and allelic heterogeneity. Most available tests are sequence-based, capable of detecting known or novel pathogenic variants in these genes. For a quick comparison of labs offering these tests, including what genes are on their panels, visit NextGxDx (nextgxdx.com).

> **Key Point**
>
> Screening athletes for sudden cardiac death genes Some high school and collegiate sports programs require participants to be screened for potential sudden cardiac death before participating in sports. Guidelines from the American College of Preventive Medicine recommend against routine genetic screening in individuals without personal risk factors[11].

Setting expectations

The yield for genetic testing varies across conditions, largely as a result of our understanding of the genetic architecture of the condition. For DCM, the yield is only about 20–30%[10]. In probable FH cases, genetic testing will be positive in about 70–80% of cases.[4] Diagnostic yield is estimated at 60–80% for LQTS and 40–60% for HCM[10]. A more recent study from an academic laboratory performed sequencing on >2900 patients with HCM for a panel of 11 genes related to HCM[12]. Their diagnostic yield was about 32%, with inconclusive results in an additional 15%. An expanded gene panel of 50 genes increased the diagnostic yield insignificantly. Genetic testing of at-risk family members was able to rule out the need for longitudinal cardiac evaluations in 691 individuals, resulting in a substantial cost savings.

Molecular autopsies of patients with sudden unexplained death can diagnose the cause of death (usually inherited channelopathies) in up to 33% of individuals[13].

PHARMACOGENOMICS

There are many drugs with pharmacogenomic information in the drug label, but not all of these are clinically valid or useful. There are three cardiovascular drugs that have a substantial body of evidence supporting the clinical validity

[4] http://www.ncbi.nlm.nih.gov/books/NBK174884/

Table 7-4. Drugs used to treat cardiovascular disease with clinically valid pharmacogenomic tests.

	Clopidogrel (Plavix)	Simvastatin (Zocor)	Warfarin (Coumadin)
Gene(s)	CYP2C19	SLCO1B1	CYP2C9/VKORC1
Drug class	Anti-platelet	Lipid lowering	Anti-coagulant
Utility	Efficacy	Toxicity (myopathy)	Proper dosing for both efficacy and toxicity (bleeding)
Effect	1.75 to 3.82-fold increased odds of stent thrombosis in poor metabolizer ACS patients undergoing PCI	2.3 to 3.2-fold increased odds of myopathy in carriers of 1 or 2 risk alleles, respectively	About 40% of dose variance explained by these two genes

ACS, acute coronary syndromes; PCI, percutaneous coronary intervention.

and utility, for which there are also dosing guidelines available (Table 7-4). However, not all of these tests are widely utilized and their coverage by insurance companies varies. The tests are most useful for initial drug or dose selection, especially when the genotype information is already available on the patient, as in the case of preemptive testing.

Clopidogrel

Patients who harbor specific variants in their CYP2C19 gene that lead to reduced activity of this drug metabolizing enzyme are classified as poor metabolizers of clopidogrel. As a result, standard doses of clopidogrel are subtherapeutic in these patients, putting them at risk of major adverse cardiovascular events and, in particular, of stent thrombosis among patients receiving drug-eluting stents[14,15]. Guidelines from the Clinical Pharmacogenomics Implementation Consortium (CPIC)[16] suggest that patients who are known CYP2C19 poor to intermediate metabolizers should consider alternate therapies, including prasugrel and ticagrelor, which are not influenced by variation in this gene (https://www.pharmgkb.org/chemical/PA449053#tabview=tab0&subtab=31). Patients who are CYP2C19 ultrarapid metabolizers (genotype *17/*17) may be at increased risk of bleeding, but the supporting clinical evidence of bleeding or adverse clinical response in these patients is not very strong.

CYP2C19 genotype is not the only factor contributing to variation in clopidogrel response. Moreover, several logistical barriers to ordering a test for CYP2C19 prevent many health care providers from using this information in drug selection or dosing.

Simvastatin

Among users of the lipid-lowering drug simvastatin, a small percentage develop muscle toxicity including myalgias, myopathy, and in rare cases the more serious and life-threatening rhabdomyolysis. These side effects can influence medication adherence. The strongest predictor of muscle toxicity in users of simvastatin is dose[17], which led the U.S. Food and Drug Administration (FDA) to recommend against an 80 mg daily starting dose. However, even at lower doses (40 mg daily), there is a risk of muscle toxicity and this risk is associated to a modest degree with a genetic variant (rs4149056) of the transporter gene *SLCO1B1*. Patients with the risk allele have a two to threefold increased odds of myopathy[19] and a threefold odds of drug discontinuation[20]. Information about *SLCO1B1* is not found in the FDA label for simvastatin, even though the relationship has been known for some time.

The relationship between *SLCO1B1* and myopathy is not seen for all statin drugs[18-20]. Guidelines from CPIC[21], found on the PharmGKB website (https://www.pharmgkb.org/chemical/PA451363#tabview=tab0&subtab=31) suggest that patients who are known to carry a *SLCO1B1* variant should be given a lower dose of the drug. If optimal efficacy is not achieved with a lower dose of simvastatin, alternate therapies should be considered.

Warfarin

Correct dosing of warfarin is essential to achieve efficacy and avoid toxicity (bleeding), and difficult to achieve given its narrow therapeutic index. Studies support that knowledge of genetic variation can help reduce side effects and increase efficacy of warfarin[22]; however, the results of several major clinical trials evaluating the clinical utility of pharmacogenomic testing for warfarin dosing were conflicting [23-25].

PharmGKB recommends that the best way to estimate the dose of warfarin is to use an algorithm from warfarindosing.org. This algorithm includes variation in two genes, *CYP2C9* and *VKORC1*, which contribute to about half of the variability in warfarin dose in Caucasians. Dosing guidelines from CPIC[26] can be found on the PharmGKB website: https://www.pharmgkb.org/chemical/PA451906.

Practice Point: Clinical Scenario

A patient has been diagnosed with familial hypercholesterolemia (FH). How do you carry out cascade screening to identify other affected relatives of the patient?

When a patient with a definitive diagnosis of FH is found to carry a pathogenic, high penetrance risk allele, it is recommended that other family members, even those that appear healthy, are screened for FH. FH is inherited in an autosomal dominant fashion, meaning that the presence of one pathogenic variant is sufficient to cause the disease. In a typical autosomal dominant disease, the variant is inherited from one parent and passed to 50% of their offspring.

Screening should include a minimum of first-degree relatives (parents, siblings, and children over 2 years). Screening may comprise measuring cholesterol levels and/or genetic testing. For genetic testing, information about the exact genetic variant found in the index case should be provided to the testing lab. The test will cost much less than the initial genetic screening test because the variant is already known.

For more information about cascade screening of FH, visit the website of the FH Foundation (https://thefhfoundation.org/familial-hypercholesterolemia-patients-should-ask-family-members-to-undergo-cascade-testing/).

RESOURCES

Exploring Predisposition and Treatment Response—The Promise of Genomics[27]

An excellent review of precision medicine in cardiovascular disease.

Evidence for Clinical Implementation of Pharmacogenomics in Cardiac Drugs[28]

A comprehensive assessment of the pharmacogenomic evidence of clinical utility for routinely used cardiovascular drugs.

Genetics and Cardiovascular Disease: A Policy Statement from the American Heart Association[29]

Guideline from the AHA providing policy recommendations regarding genetic testing as it relates to personal and family history, examination, counseling, and impact of the practice of cardiovascular medicine and research.

U.S. Guidelines Addressing Genetic Testing for Hypertrophic Cardiomyopathy

2011 guideline for the diagnosis and treatment of hypertrophiccardiomyopathy from the AHA/ACCF.

American College of Cardiology Foundation—Medical Specialty Society; American Heart Association—Professional Association.

European Guidelines Addressing Genetic Testing for Channelopathies And Cardiomyopathies

2011 expert consensus statement on the state of genetic testing for the channelopathies and cardiomyopathies from the HRS/EHRA.

European Heart Rhythm Association—Professional Association; Heart Rhythm Society—Professional Association.

REFERENCES

1. Roberts R, Stewart AF. Genes and coronary artery disease: where are we? *J Am Coll Cardiol.* 2012;60:1715-1721.
2. Evaluation of Genomic Applications in Practice and Prevention (EGAPP) Working Group. Recommendations from the EGAPP Working Group: genomic profiling to assess cardiovascular risk to improve cardiovascular health. *Genet Med.* 2010;12:839-843.
3. Goldstein BA, Knowles JW, Salfati E, Ioannidis JP, Assimes TL. Simple, standardized incorporation of genetic risk into non-genetic risk prediction tools for complex traits: coronary heart disease as an example. *Front Genet.* 2014;5:254.
4. Gersh BJ, Maron BJ, Bonow RO, et al. 2011 ACCF/AHA guideline for the diagnosis and treatment of hypertrophic cardiomyopathy: a report of the American College of Cardiology Foundation/American Heart Association Task Force on Practice Guidelines. *Circulation.* 2011;124:e783-e831.
5. Nordestgaard BG, Chapman MJ, Humphries SE, et al. Familial hypercholesterolaemia is underdiagnosed and undertreated in the general population: guidance for clinicians to prevent coronary heart disease: consensus statement of the European Atherosclerosis Society. *Eur Heart J.* 2013;34:3478-3490.
6. Starr B, Hadfield SG, Hutten BA, et al. Development of sensitive and specific age- and gender-specific low-density lipoprotein cholesterol cutoffs for diagnosis of first-degree relatives with familial hypercholesterolaemia in cascade testing. *Clin Chem Lab Med.* 2008;46:791-803.
7. Gohil R, Peck G, Sharma P. The genetics of venous thromboembolism. A meta-analysis involving approximately 120,000 cases and 180,000 controls. *Thromb Haemost.* 2009;102:360-370.
8. Chang MH, Lindegren ML, Butler MA, et al. Prevalence in the United States of selected candidate gene variants: Third National Health and Nutrition Examination Survey, 1991-1994. *Am J Epidemiol.* 2009;169:54-66.
9. Van Driest SL, Wells QS, Stallings S, et al. Association of arrhythmia-related genetic variants with phenotypes documented in electronic medical records. *JAMA.* 2016;315:47-57.
10. Ackerman MJ, Priori SG, Willems S, et al. HRS/EHRA expert consensus statement on the state of genetic testing for the channelopathies and cardiomyopathies: this document was developed as a partnership between the Heart Rhythm Society (HRS) and the European Heart Rhythm Association (EHRA). *Heart Rhythm.* 2011;8:1308-1339.
11. Mahmood S, Lim L, Akram Y, Alford-Morales S, Sherin K, Committee APP. Screening for sudden cardiac death before participation in high school and collegiate sports: American College of Preventive Medicine position statement on preventive practice. *Am J Prev Med.* 2013;45:130-133.
12. Alfares AA, Kelly MA, McDermott G, et al. Results of clinical genetic testing of 2,912 probands with hypertrophic cardiomyopathy: expanded panels offer limited additional sensitivity. *Genet Med.* 2015;17:880-888.
13. Semsarian C, Hamilton RM. Key role of the molecular autopsy in sudden unexpected death. *Heart Rhythm.* 2012;9:145-150.
14. Hulot JS, Collet JP, Silvain J, et al. Cardiovascular risk in clopidogrel-treated patients according to cytochrome P450 2C19*2 loss-of-function allele or proton pump inhibitor coadministration: a systematic meta-analysis. *J Am Coll Cardiol.* 2010;56:134-143.
15. Mega JL, Simon T, Collet JP, et al. Reduced-function CYP2C19 genotype and risk of adverse clinical outcomes among patients treated with clopidogrel predominantly for PCI: a meta-analysis. *JAMA.* 2010;304:1821-1830.
16. Scott SA, Sangkuhl K, Stein CM, et al. Clinical Pharmacogenetics Implementation Consortium guidelines for CYP2C19 genotype and clopidogrel therapy: 2013 update. *Clin Pharmacol Ther.* 2013;94:317-323.
17. SEARCH Collaborative Group, Link E, Parish S, et al. SLCO1B1 variants and statin-induced myopathy—a genomewide study. *N Engl J Med.* 2008;359:789-799.
18. Brunham LR, Lansberg PJ, Zhang L, et al. Differential effect of the rs4149056 variant in SLCO1B1 on myopathy associated with simvastatin and atorvastatin. *Pharmacogenomics J.* 2012;12:233-237.

19. Voora D, Shah SH, Spasojevic I, et al. The SLCO1B1*5 genetic variant is associated with statin-induced side effects. *J Am Coll Cardiol.* 2009;54:1609-1616.
20. Puccetti L, Ciani F, Auteri A. Genetic involvement in statins induced myopathy. Preliminary data from an observational case-control study. *Atherosclerosis.* 2010;211:28-29.
21. Wilke RA, Ramsey LB, Johnson SG, et al. The clinical pharmacogenomics implementation consortium: CPIC guideline for SLCO1B1 and simvastatin-induced myopathy. *Clin Pharmacol Ther.* 2012;92:112-117.
22. Epstein RS, Moyer TP, Aubert RE, et al. Warfarin genotyping reduces hospitalization rates results from the MM-WES (Medco-Mayo Warfarin Effectiveness study). *J Am Coll Cardiol.* 2010;55:2804-2812.
23. Kimmel SE, French B, Kasner SE, et al. A pharmacogenetic versus a clinical algorithm for warfarin dosing. *N Engl J Med.* 2013;369:2283-2293.
24. Pirmohamed M, Burnside G, Eriksson N, et al. A randomized trial of genotype-guided dosing of warfarin. *N Engl J Med.* 2013;369:2294-2303.
25. Verhoef TI, Ragia G, de Boer A, et al. A randomized trial of genotype-guided dosing of acenocoumarol and phenprocoumon. *N Engl J Med.* 2013;369:2304-2312.
26. Johnson JA, Gong L, Whirl-Carrillo M, et al. Clinical Pharmacogenetics Implementation Consortium guidelines for CYP2C9 and VKORC1 genotypes and warfarin dosing. *Clin Pharmacol Ther.* 2011;90:625-629.
27. Pan S, Knowles JW. Exploring predisposition and treatment response—the promise of genomics. *Prog Cardiovasc Dis.* 2012;55:56-63.
28. Kaufman AL, Spitz J, Jacobs M, et al. Evidence for clinical implementation of pharmacogenomics in cardiac drugs. *Mayo Clin Proc.* 2015;90:716-729.
29. Ashley EA, Hershberger RE, Caleshu C, et al. Genetics and cardiovascular disease: a policy statement from the American Heart Association. *Circulation.* 2012;126:142-157.

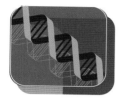

CHAPTER 8

Cancer Predisposition Testing

The availability and general awareness of hereditary cancer predisposition tests has grown substantially in the past several years, owing in part to the continued discovery of cancer susceptibility genes, the reversal of gene patent laws[1], and high-profile celebrity cases[2]. The result is that numerous laboratories now offer genetic tests for inherited breast, colorectal, and other cancers. The types of tests offered is changing as well, due to the introduction of next-generation sequencing technologies, which allow for faster and cheaper analysis of genetic variation. The field is moving away from testing single genes and toward testing panels of genes. Recently, we have seen a nearly 10-fold drop in the cost of genetic testing[3]. Patients with a personal or family history of cancer may be candidates for inherited cancer predisposition testing, and in time with fewer barriers to access, screening for cancer risk may spread to the general population.

FAMILIAL RISK OF CANCER

Cancer is typically a late onset disease, which appears in some cases to cluster in families. For frequently occurring cancers like prostate, lung, colon, breast, and bladder, the risk to siblings of an affected patient is about two- to fourfold increased[4]. Familial risk may reflect an inherited predisposition to cancer, but may also simply be a sign of shared environment or chance (larger families will have higher chance of a family history of cancer). The majority of cancer cases (90%) occur sporadically, the result of environment or intrinsic biological factors. Up to 10% of cancer is thought to be heritable, but the genetic basis of that heritability is complex. Much of the heritability probably reflects the combined effects of numerous low-risk variants and complex gene by environment interactions, but high-risk Mendelian (single gene) forms of cancer exist as well.

GENETIC BASIS OF FAMILIAL CANCERS

The genetic architecture of cancers is complex and only partially understood. About half of the genetic basis of familial cancers remains unexplained, leaving family history remaining as an important risk factor for some cancers. The genetic basis of breast cancer is illustrated in Figure 8-1. There are dozens of common low-penetrance genetic variants that have been robustly associated with breast cancer, but each contributing only a

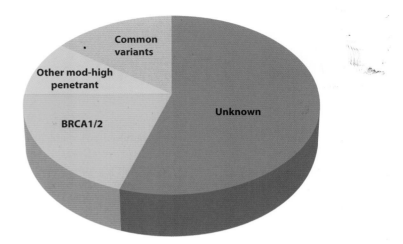

Figure 8-1. **The genetic basis of breast cancer.** Five to ten percent of breast cancer is thought to be hereditary, but the genetic basis of only about half of that is understood and consists of moderate to high penetrance gene variants (*BRCA1/2* and other genes) and common variants of small effect.

very small increase in risk. These common variants do not make good predictive genetic tests.

The genetic basis of breast cancer also includes two main, highly penetrant (high risk) genes, *BRCA1* and *BRCA2*, which account for about half of hereditary breast cancer. There are also a handful of other moderate to highly penetrant genes (e.g., *PTEN*, *ATM*, *TP53*) known to cause familial cancer syndromes that include breast cancer as one of the features. For these high- and moderate-penetrance genes, genetic testing is available.

CLINICAL FEATURES OF HEREDITARY CANCERS

While family history of cancer is often the motivation for pursuing genetic testing, not all familial cancer is due to a single, moderate- to high-risk gene. One of the challenges with hereditary cancer is that, at the histopathological level, it may be indistinguishable from the more common, sporadic form of that cancer. However, there are a few telltale signs of hereditary cancer, including the following:

- Family history—especially multigenerational, in first-degree relatives. Also, multiple family members with a rare type of cancer (e.g., cancer of the fallopian tube).

- Earlier age of onset than is typical for that cancer. Of note, approximately 8% of cancers appearing in children are associated with an inherited syndrome[5].

- Clinical presentation (even in absence of family history)
- Multiple independent different types of cancer in same person
- Bilateral, occurring in both of a pair of organs (i.e., both kidneys or both breasts)
- Unusual cases (e.g., male breast cancer)
- More detailed, cancer-specific referral indications for predisposition testing are outlined in a recent guidance from the American College of Medical Genetics and Genomics (ACMG) and the National Society of Genetic Counselors (NSGC)[6].

> **Key Point:**
>
> One of the greatest misconceptions about hereditary breast and ovarian cancers is that they can't be inherited from a male. It's true that males don't themselves develop ovarian cancer and it's rare that they develop breast cancer. However, whether they can or can't develop these cancers themselves, they can indeed carry predisposing mutations and pass them down to their offspring.

How to select the right test for cancer predisposition

There are a number of good predictive genetic predisposition tests for hereditary cancer syndromes (Table 8-1). These syndromes are characterized by variable expression of cancer in mutation carriers. In other words, each mutation carrier, even in the same family, can develop a different type of cancer and at different ages. Nonetheless, each syndrome has a recognizable pattern of cancers that is typical.

There are many choices of laboratories and tests, mostly gene-sequencing panels, for inherited cancers. Gene panels for hereditary breast cancer testing, for example, range in size from a few to several dozen genes. See Appendix 5 for more guidance on selecting a laboratory and test.

Who should get tested?

Guidelines from the National Comprehensive Cancer Network (NCCN) and others recognize the value of genetic testing in providing a possible explanation for a patient's personal or family history of cancer (see Resources section). More information about collecting family history can be found in Appendix 4. Briefly, a family history should include information about the type of cancer, age of onset, family relationship, and any unusual features.

Patients with a personal history of cancer may wish to be tested in order to determine if their cancer is hereditary, with possible implications for their own risk of additional cancers, as well as risk to their family members. More often, in the primary care setting, patients with a family history, and no personal history, of cancer may wish to be tested to determine their risk. In the latter case, efforts should be made to have affected family members tested first, as knowledge of a specific genetic variant in the affected person can improve genetic test interpretation in the person being tested.

Individuals at greatly increased risk of developing cancer due to inherited predisposition have several preventive care options including screening and surgical and therapeutic prophylaxis. Detailed information about

Table 8-1. List of most common cancer syndromes with available genetic tests and the different cancers that mutation carriers are known to develop (note: risk of each type of cancer is not the same).

Cancer syndrome	Genes	Related cancers
Hereditary breast and ovarian cancer syndrome	BRCA1, BRCA2	Female breast, ovarian, prostate, pancreatic, and male breast cancer
Lynch syndrome (hereditary nonpolyposis colorectal cancer)	MSH2, MLH1, MSH6, PMS2, EPCAM	Colorectal, endometrial, ovarian, renal pelvis, pancreatic, small intestine, liver and biliary tract, stomach, brain, and breast cancers
Familial adenomatous polyposis	APC	Colorectal cancer, multiple nonmalignant colon polyps, and both noncancerous (benign) and cancerous tumors in the small intestine, brain, stomach, bone, skin, and other tissues
Li–Fraumeni syndrome	TP53	Breast cancer, soft tissue sarcoma, osteosarcoma (bone cancer), leukemia, brain tumors, adrenocortical carcinoma (cancer of the adrenal glands), and other cancers
Cowden syndrome	PTEN	Breast, thyroid, endometrial (uterine lining), and other cancers
Retinoblastoma	RB1	Eye cancer (cancer of the retina), pinealoma (cancer of the pineal gland), osteosarcoma, melanoma, and soft tissue sarcoma
Wermer syndrome (multiple endocrine neoplasia type 1)	MEN1	Parathyroid (usually benign), pituitary gland, and pancreatic endocrine tumors
Multiple endocrine neoplasia type 2	RET	Medullary thyroid cancer and pheochromocytoma (benign adrenal gland tumor)
Von Hippel–Lindau syndrome	VHL	Kidney, brain, spinal cord, adrenal gland, retina and multiple nonmalignant tumors, including pheochromocytoma

management of mutation carriers for various hereditary cancer syndromes can be found at GeneReviews.[1]

Current testing recommendations are limited to individuals with suspected hereditary cancer as evidenced by a strong family history. More recent research in the area of breast cancer suggests that limiting testing to those with a family history will miss a substantial portion of mutation carriers[7]. Based on these findings and the fact that testing is becoming more accessible, some have called for widespread population-based breast cancer predisposition screening of women beginning at age 30[8]. However, population-wide screening comes with possible financial and health risks, due to ambiguous test results, at least initially. The hope is that over time, with testing of large numbers of women, both with and without cancer, we will learn more about

[1] http://www.ncbi.nlm.nih.gov/books/NBK1116/

the true penetrance and pathogenicity of variants. Screening for hereditary cancers can never replace common sense interventions to reduce the risk of cancer, such as refraining from smoking, adopting healthy dietary and exercise habits, sun protection, and currently recommended screening protocols (e.g., mammogram, colonoscopy).

Understanding results from cancer predisposition tests

Based on our experience, a typical cancer gene panel will reveal approximately two to three protein-coding variants per gene per patient. Half of these will be obviously benign, while the others will require careful interpretation by the testing laboratory. To learn more about how laboratories interpret and classify variants, see Appendix 6.

Positive Results

Positive results, where a patient carries a pathogenic variant in a cancer predisposing gene, need to be carefully communicated to the patient so that they understand the risk of cancer to themselves and their family members, and the options available to mitigate their risk. Engaging with a genetic counselor is a good idea, as they can help the patient understand the results, provide supportive counseling, and help patients communicate genetic test results with other family members.

Negative results

Negative results, where a patient only carries benign variants, or no variants at all in the cancer predisposing genes, needs to be carefully communicated as well. Most cancer is not inherited meaning the patient is still at risk for sporadic cancer, but their risk is no greater than the average population. A patient with a strong family history who tests negative still has a risk of cancer that is *increased* above the average population since we currently don't know all of the genes underlying hereditary cancer.

Managing expectations

A report from one commercial lab found that among 10,000 patients with breast, ovarian, or colon/stomach cancer tested with one of eight multigene panels comprising combinations of 29 genes, the diagnostic yield was 9.7, 13.4, and 14.8%, respectively[9]. Approximately half of the pathogenic variants identified in patients with breast or ovarian cancer were in genes other than *BRCA1/2*.

Variants of uncertain significance

The biggest challenge in interpreting genetic testing results is understanding and communicating variants of uncertain significance (VUS). These indeterminate results can cause distress in patients and drive some to consider potentially dangerous and unnecessary prophylactic surgery[10]. Estimates of the rate of identifying VUS vary by population, by gene, and by testing laboratory. Laboratories with more experience and volume of testing may have lower VUS rates due to their cumulative knowledge. VUS rates will decline over time as more testing is performed and results shared with the medical community.

The uncertainty with a VUS may stem from a lack of prior observation of this variant and/or lack of clinical or functional evidence supporting a role of the variant in cancer. About 10% of variants observed in cancer gene panels are novel, having not been previously observed in cancer patients or the general population. Clinical and functional evidence is not always available, even for previously observed variants and it is not customary for laboratories to pursue such studies on variants uncovered during routine testing. The prior probability that a VUS will be pathogenic is less than 10%[11].

In our experience, the best way to reduce the negative impact of a VUS result is to counsel the patient about this eventuality *before* the test is sent. Explaining that the results are not always binary (positive vs. negative) but include an uncertain middle ground, will help prepare the patient and, in situations where the patient is a questionable candidate for testing, may allow the patient to pause and consider further before moving forward.

A patient with a VUS may benefit from having other family members, both affected and unaffected, tested to determine if the variant cosegregates with cancer in their family. This information may be useful for further interpretation of the variant. Family studies must be interpreted with caution, because an unaffected relative with a variant may simply not have developed cancer yet, and an affected relative may in fact have a sporadic cancer. Currently there are not any options available to order follow-up functional studies of a variant, except in the research setting.

Practice Point: Clinical Scenario 1

Communicating positive test results to family members: A patient with a strong family history of colorectal and other cancers undergoes testing and is found to carry a pathogenic mutation in MLH1, a known high-risk gene for Lynch syndrome. They are wondering what, if anything, to tell their siblings and other family members about their test results.

Patients who undergo hereditary cancer testing may choose to share test results, both positive and negative, with other adult family members because the results may inform the family members' risk of cancer as well. Information about the specific gene(s) tested and the specific gene mutation found (if positive) should be conveyed to the family member, and they should be encouraged to discuss any positive results with their doctor and/or a genetic counselor. Testing family members, if desired, is expedited by knowledge of the precise gene and mutation in the family.

(Continued)

It may be helpful to provide patients with literature explaining hereditary cancer testing. Literature may be obtained from the website of the testing laboratory, or from any of a number of reputable websites found in the Resource section below. This literature can be shared with the patients' family members and serve as an entrée into discussing their own testing options.

Family members should be given the opportunity to make an informed, personal decision about whether they will undergo testing themselves. More information about sharing results with family members can be found at Cancer.net (http://www.cancer.net/navigating-cancer-care/cancer-basics/genetics/sharing-genetic-test-results-your-family).

Practice Point: Clinical Scenario 2

Communicating VUS results to a patient: A patient has undergone cancer gene panel testing because of a family history of brain tumors. The results come back with a VUS in PMS2, a gene for Lynch syndrome where brain cancer is one of the features. How should this result be interpreted and communicated to the patient?

The important points to make to the patient are the following:

1. The average person has approximately 4 million variants in their genome, but not all of them are bad. In fact, only a small portion of variants may be affecting a person's health. Similarly, it is normal for a person to have several variants in cancer genes, but not all of them will lead to cancer.
2. A VUS lacks sufficient evidence to declare that it is disease causing or benign. Therefore, this information alone should not be used to guide health decisions.
3. The laboratory will continue to monitor and update the variant classification as more data become available and many labs will issue an update if/when those changes occur. To facilitate this, physicians, other providers, and patients should periodically request updates on the status of VUS reclassification and remain in contact with each other.
4. Consider having other family members tested to determine whether the variant is present in other family members, even those unaffected, and whether those members with the variant have cancer or not.

Practice Point: Clinical Scenario 3

Whom to test? A healthy young woman's older sister was just diagnosed with breast cancer. She would like to undergo testing of known breast cancer genes to learn if she is at heightened risk for having breast cancer herself. How best to proceed?

The optimal next step is to determine if the sister with cancer has had genetic testing. If a pathogenic mutation is detected in the affected sister it is straightforward to determine its presence or absence in the healthy sister. If no mutations are found, testing the healthy sister becomes unnecessary.

If the sister with cancer cannot be tested for some reason (e.g., through lack of desire or access), then it is reasonable to test the healthy sister, particularly if the affected sister had a red flag such as cancer at an atypically young age or bilateral cancer. However, if no pathogenic variants are identified, the healthy sister cannot be confident that she is not at an increased risk of cancer. Family history remains important. If a mutation is later identified in the healthy patient's sister, the healthy patient's negative result is then more reassuring.

RESOURCES

ASCO Genetic testing toolkit (http://www.asco.org/genetics-toolkit/welcome)

The purpose of this toolkit is to provide oncology professionals with the tools and resources that will assist them in effectively integrating hereditary cancer risk assessment into practice.

NCI hereditary cancer fact sheet (http://www.cancer.gov/cancertopics/genetics/genetic-testing-fact-sheet)

Learn the what, who, and how of genetic testing for cancer from the U.S. National Cancer Institutes.

Guidelines

General resource for guidelines for genetic testing from CDC OPHG (http://www.cdc.gov/genomics/gtesting/tier.htm)

General resource for guidelines for genetic testing from the U.S. Centers for Disease Control and Prevention, Office of Public Health Genomics.

Various cancer practice guidelines from National Society of Genetic Counselors (NSGC) (http://nsgc.org/p/cm/ld/fid=70)

Various cancer practice guidelines from National Society of Genetic Counselors.

ASCO familial cancer screening (http://jco.ascopubs.org/content/early/2015/08/31/JCO.2015.63.0996.full)

Familial cancer screening guidelines from the American Society of Clinical Oncology.

NCCN breast/ovarian genetic screening (http://www.nccn.org/professionals/physician_gls/pdf/genetics_screening.pdf)

Breast/ovarian genetic screening guidelines from the National Comprehensive Cancer Network.

NCCN colorectal genetic screening (http://www.nccn.org/professionals/physician_gls/pdf/genetics_colon.pdf)

Colorectal genetic screening guidelines from the National Comprehensive Cancer Network.

REFERENCES

1. Sherkow JS, Greely HT. The history of patenting genetic material. *Annu Rev Genet.* 2015;49:161-182.
2. Lebo PB, Quehenberger F, Kamolz LP, Lumenta DB. The Angelina effect revisited: exploring a media-related impact on public awareness. *Cancer.* 2015;121:3959-3964.
3. Clain E, Trosman JR, Douglas MP, Weldon CB, Phillips KA. Availability and payer coverage of BRCA1/2 tests and gene panels. *Nat Biotechnol.* 2015;33:900-902.
4. Mucci LA, Hjelmborg JB, Harris JR, et al. Familial risk and heritability of cancer among twins in Nordic countries. *JAMA.* 2016;315:68-76.
5. Zhang J, Walsh MF, Wu G, et al. Germline mutations in predisposition genes in pediatric cancer. *N Engl J Med.* 2015;373:2336-2346.
6. Hampel H, Bennett RL, Buchanan A, et al. A practice guideline from the American College of Medical Genetics and Genomics and the National Society of Genetic Counselors: referral indications for cancer predisposition assessment. *Genet Med.* 2015;17:70-87.
7. Gabai-Kapara E, Lahad A, Kaufman B, et al. Population-based screening for breast and ovarian cancer risk due to BRCA1 and BRCA2. *Proc Natl Acad Sci US A.* 2014;111:14205-14210.
8. King MC, Levy-Lahad E, Lahad A. Population-based screening for BRCA1 and BRCA2: 2014 Lasker Award. *JAMA.* 2014;312:1091-1092.
9. Susswein LR, Marshall ML, Nusbaum R, et al. Pathogenic and likely pathogenic variant prevalence among the first 10,000 patients referred for next-generation cancer panel testing. *Genet Med.* 2015.
10. Murray ML, Cerrato F, Bennett RL, Jarvik GP. Follow-up of carriers of BRCA1 and BRCA2 variants of unknown significance: variant reclassification and surgical decisions. *Genet Med.* 2011;13:998-1005.
11. Goldgar DE, Easton DF, Deffenbaugh AM, et al. Integrated evaluation of DNA sequence variants of unknown clinical significance: application to BRCA1 and BRCA2. *Am J Hum Genet.* 2004;75:535-544.

CHAPTER 9

Genomic Guided Cancer Treatment Decisions

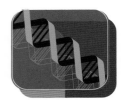

Precision medicine is making a big impact on how we define and treat cancers. Sequencing the tumors of thousands of cancer patients has revealed the molecular landscape of this disease. From this vast trove of molecular data, novel drug targets have emerged, along with molecular profiles of drug efficacy. According to a 2015 report from the Personalized Medicine Coalition, 73% of oncology drugs in development are personalized medicines.[1] The classification of cancer is changing from being based primarily on tissue of origin or appearance under a microscope to a classification based on a tumor's molecular signature. Health care providers should be aware of these changes and how personalized cancer therapies offer expanded treatment options for their patients.

CANCER GENOMICS

Normal cellular growth (cell division or mitosis) is controlled by cell cycle regulators, growth inhibitors (tumor suppressors), growth factors (oncogenes), growth factor receptors, and other molecules. Cancerous cells have acquired the ability to bypass growth signaling and lose growth control. Cancer is usually the result of a cascade of mutations in key pathways regulating cell division that have accumulated in a given cell over decades. These **somatic** DNA variants differ from **germline** DNA variants in that they are not present in all of the cells in the body, only the cancerous cells, and are not inherited. These mutations are acquired through faulty DNA damage repair or during normal replication. The cancerous cell then divides uncontrollably and the resulting tumor invades the surrounding tissue and frequently metastasizes. Understanding the key molecular drivers of cancer progression has helped us develop targeted treatments that act on these root molecular causes of cancer.

At the molecular level, tumors are characterized by a wide range of mutation types (Fig. 9-1)[1]. The most common are single-base substitutions (SBS), but larger variations in the form of insertion/deletion of a few nucleotides (InDels, amplifications, larger deletions, and translocations) are also

---

[1] http://www.personalizedmedicinecoalition.org/Userfiles/PMC-Corporate/file/PMC_2015_annual_report.pdf

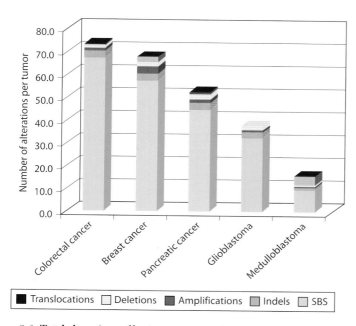

Figure 9-1. Total alterations affecting protein-coding genes in selected tumors
(Reproduced with permission from Vogelstein B, Papadopoulos N, Velculescu VE, et al:
Cancer genome landscapes, Science. 2013 Mar 29;339(6127):1546-5158).

Average number and types of genomic alterations per tumor, including single-base
substitutions (SBS), small insertions and deletions (InDels), amplifications, and
homozygous deletions, as determined by genome-wide sequencing studies. For
colorectal, breast, and pancreatic ductal cancer, and medulloblastomas, translocations are also included.

present. There are over 500 genes for which somatic mutations have been
causally implicated in cancer (http://cancer.sanger.ac.uk/census/) and others undoubtedly remain to be discovered. The average solid tumor has 33–66
mutated genes[1], the spectrum and number of which varies by cancer type.
Childhood tumors tend to have fewer mutations than adult-onset cancers.
Some tumors have characteristic mutation signatures based on different mutational processes, like exposure to cigarette smoke[2].

The key to understanding the molecular underpinnings of cancer is dis-
tinguishing the mutations driving cancer development from those that are
mere passengers. Known mechanisms of cancer drivers include activation of
oncogenes, inactivation of DNA repair enzymes, deactivation of tumor suppressors, and modification of chromatin. Some but not all classes of cancer
drivers may be amenable to therapeutic modulation. For example, the deactivation of a tumor suppressor is difficult to therapeutically reactivate. In contrast, activated oncogenes are often targeted with monoclonal antibodies or

small molecules, which deactivate these cancer-causing pathways. The spectrum of cancer drivers within a given tumor type reveals the heterogeneous nature of cancer[3]. For example, what we once defined as melanoma is now recognized as BRAF-positive or BRAF-negative melanoma, a meaningful distinction with respect to treatment. In time, it is expected that cancers will be defined by their molecular profile rather than their issue of origin.

IMPACT OF TUMOR MOLECULAR PROFILING ON CLINICAL MANAGEMENT

Tumor molecular profiling, for the purpose of this discussion, refers to testing a sample of the tumor for presence of one or more molecular alterations that may be useful for guiding treatment decisions. These alterations may include changes in the tumor at the level of DNA, RNA, or protein. There are several applications of tumor profiling.

- There are multianalyte gene expression profiles for determining the likelihood of cancer recurrence. These are used to inform the timing and type of treatment.
- Tumor profiling is used for selecting the most efficacious therapy for a patient based on presence of specific alterations in the tumor. These profiles may consist of targeted analysis of specific variation (i.e., *BRAF* point mutations or *HER2* gene amplification) used as a companion diagnostic for a U.S. Food and Drug Administration (FDA)-approved therapy or a more broad assessment of alterations in panels of genes for the purpose of identifying additional treatment options.
- Tumor profiling can also better define the tissue origin of a tumor or determine if a tumor is a new primary versus a recurrence of a past cancer.

Cancer recurrence risk profiles

Several tests are marketed for the purpose of assessing the likelihood of cancer recurrence or aggressiveness (Table 9-1), especially in the area of breast cancer[4]. These multianalyte algorithm-based assays are based on simultaneous measurement of expression of dozens of genes in a tumor sample and are typically used in conjunction with standard clinicopathological parameters to provide each patient with a recurrence risk score. The tests vary according to whether they predict early or late recurrence, and may only be valid in certain patient subpopulations. Risk of recurrence may be used to determine whether to treat patients early or watch and wait.

Targeted treatments—Companion diagnostics

Targeted treatments are those that are designed to modulate specific cancer driver genes, or targets, many of which are oncogenic targets that are *activated* in tumor cells, but not in healthy tissue. Activation can be triggered

Table 9-1. Tumor profiling tests for determining cancer recurrence risk.

Vendor	Test	Cancer	Medicare coverage?
Genomic Health	Oncotype Dx®	Breast	Yes
Genomic Health	Oncotype Dx®	Colon	Yes
Agendia	Mammaprint®	Breast	Yes
Myriad Genetics	MyPlan™	Lung	
Myriad Genetics	MyPath®	Melanoma	
Myriad Genetics	Prolaris®	Prostate	
Myriad Genetics	Endopredict®	Breast	
NanoString Technologies	Prosigna™ Breast Cancer Prognostic Gene Signature Assay (formerly PAM50)	Breast	
Biotheranostics	Breast Cancer Index℠	Breast	

by mutation or epigenetic factors and can affect the drug target directly, or genes in the drug pathway. Molecular tumor profiling can be used to predict tumor sensitivity or resistance to these FDA-approved targeted therapies. These therapies are typically codeveloped with a companion diagnostic test for relevant target alterations in the tumor. A list of FDA-approved companion diagnostics can be found on the FDA website.[2] Prior to prescribing the targeted therapy, the patient's tumor is tested for presence of the molecular alteration. The following examples showcase successful treatment strategies based on tumor molecular targets:

- *Breast cancer—HER2 overexpression or amplification*
  The HER2 protein is expressed at higher than normal levels in 20% of breast cancers, usually due to increase in copy number of the *HER2/neu* gene, which causes increased signal pathway activation. Herceptin® (trastuzumab) is a monoclonal antibody that binds to HER2, preventing the receptor from activating the pathways that promote the proliferation and survival of breast cancer cells.

- *Non-small cell lung carcinoma (NSCLC)—EGFR activating variants*
  Point mutations in genes can also be activating, as is the case with variants in EGFR, a protein that stimulates protein tyrosine kinase and leads

[2] http://www.fda.gov/medicaldevices/productsandmedicalprocedures/invitrodiagnostics/ucm301431.htm

to activation of downstream signaling pathways linked to cell growth. About 20% of NSCLC tumors have *EGFR* mutations that increase the kinase activity of EGFR. The majority of these mutations are either a specific SBS leading to an amino acid change (L858R) or a deletion of exon 19. Patients with these mutations are sensitive to treatment with tyrosine kinase inhibitors, with response rates of >70% in patients treated with either erlotinib or gefitinib.

• *Chronic myelogenous leukemia (CML)—BCR-ABL translocation*
Structural variants, such as translocations, can lead to fusion proteins that are activating. CML is a blood cancer caused by a reciprocal translocation (known as the Philadelphia chromosome), resulting in oncogenic *BCR-ABL* gene fusion. This translocation is found in 95% of CML. Multiple targeted ABL kinase inhibitors have been created that specifically inhibit this oncogene (imatinib, dasatinib, nilotinib). Prior to the availability of these treatments, median survival time for CML patients was only 4 years. Now, treatment extends survival to 20–25 years.

In some cases, a molecular tumor marker other than the tumor target itself can inform efficacy of the drug, offering prognostic utility. For example, some molecular markers of efficacy/response are in downstream pathway genes.

• *Colorectal cancer—KRAS mutations*
Cetuximab and panitumumab are two EGFR inhibitor antibodies used to treat colon cancer. These drugs are not efficacious for all patients. Efficacy has been linked to the presence of a genetic mutation in a downstream pathway gene, *KRAS*, found in approximately 35–40% of colorectal tumors. Tumors harboring *KRAS* mutations are not responsive to EGFR inhibition with these drugs and thus patients with these mutations are unlikely to benefit from the therapy. Companion Dx tests are available for mutations in codons 12 or 13, where most of the known deleterious mutations are known to occur.

Dozens of FDA-approved targeted treatments on the market require tumor molecular profiling, in most cases analysis of a single molecular alteration, to determine who will or will not benefit from the therapy (Table 9-2).

Tumor profiling for expanded treatment options

For some patients, knowledge of mutations in their tumor may suggest additional treatment options beyond the standard of care. One of these treatment options is off-label use of a targeted therapy approved by the FDA for a different tumor type. The rationale for this approach stems from the observation that there are some genes that are recurrently mutated in different cancers. For example, three of the most common recurrently mutated genes are *BRAF*, *PIK3CA*, and *TP53* (Fig. 9-2)[5]. Off-label use is based on

Table 9-2. FDA-approved targeted treatments currently available in the market.[a]

Cancer type	Targeted treatment
Basal cell carcinoma	Vismodegib (Erivedge™)
Brain cancer	Bevacizumab (Avastin®), everolimus (Afinitor®)
Breast cancer	Everolimus (Afinitor®), tamoxifen, toremifene (Fareston®), Trastuzumab (Herceptin®), fulvestrant (Faslodex®), anastrozole (Arimidex®), exemestane (Aromasin®), lapatinib (Tykerb®), letrozole (Femara®), pertuzumab (Perjeta™), ado-trastuzumab emtansine (Kadcyla™)
Cervical cancer	Bevacizumab (Avastin®)
Colorectal cancer	Cetuximab (Erbitux®), panitumumab (Vectibix®), bevacizumab (Avastin®), ziv-aflibercept (Zaltrap®), regorafenib (Stivarga®)
Dermatofibrosarcoma protuberans	Imatinib mesylate (Gleevec®)
Endocrine/neuroendocrine tumors	Lanreotide acetate (Somatuline® Depot)
Gastrointestinal stromal tumor	Imatinib mesylate (Gleevec®), sunitinib (Sutent®), regorafenib (Stivarga®)
Giant cell tumor of the bone	Denosumab (Xgeva®)
Head and neck cancer	Cetuximab (Erbitux®)
Kaposi sarcoma	Alitretinoin (Panretin®)
Kidney cancer	Bevacizumab (Avastin®), sorafenib (Nexavar®), sunitinib (Sutent®), pazopanib (Votrient®), temsirolimus (Torisel®), everolimus (Afinitor®), axitinib (Inlyta®)
Leukemia	Tretinoin (Vesanoid®), imatinib mesylate (Gleevec®), dasatinib (Sprycel®), nilotinib (Tasigna®), bosutinib (Bosulif®), rituximab (Rituxan®), alemtuzumab (Campath®), ofatumumab (Arzerra®), obinutuzumab (Gazyva™), ibrutinib (Imbruvica™), idelalisib (Zydelig®), blinatumomab (Blincyto™)
Liver cancer	Sorafenib (Nexavar®)
Lung cancer	Bevacizumab (Avastin®), crizotinib (Xalkori®), erlotinib (Tarceva®), gefitinib (Iressa®), afatinib dimaleate (Gilotrif®), ceritinib (LDK378/Zykadia), ramucirumab (Cyramza™)
Lymphoma	Ibritumomab tiuxetan (Zevalin®), denileukin diftitox (Ontak®), brentuximab vedotin (Adcetris®), rituximab (Rituxan®), vorinostat (Zolinza®), romidepsin (Istodax®), bexarotene (Targretin®), bortezomib (Velcade®), pralatrexate (Folotyn®), lenaliomide (Revlimid®), ibrutinib (Imbruvica™), siltuximab (Sylvant™), idelalisib (Zydelig®), belinostat (Beleodaq™)
Melanoma	Ipilimumab (Yervoy®), vemurafenib (Zelboraf®), trametinib (Mekinist®), dabrafenib (Tafinlar®), pembrolizumab (Keytruda®), nivolumab (Opdivo®)
Multiple myeloma	Bortezomib (Velcade®), carfilzomib (Kyprolis®), lenaliomide (Revlimid®), pomalidomide (Pomalyst®)
Myelodysplastic/myeloproliferative disorders	Imatinib mesylate (Gleevec®), ruxolitinib phosphate (Jakafi™)

(Continued)

Table 9-2. Continued

Cancer type	Targeted treatment
Ovarian /fallopian tube/peritoneal cancers	Bevacizumab (Avastin®), olaparib (Lynparza™)
Pancreatic cancer	Erlotinib (Tarceva®), everolimus (Afinitor®), sunitinib (Sutent®)
Prostate cancer	Cabazitaxel (Jevtana®), enzalutamide (Xtandi®), abiraterone acetate (Zytiga®), radium 223 chloride (Xofigo®)
Soft tissue sarcoma	Pazopanib (Votrient®)
Stomach or gastroesophageal junction	Trastuzumab (Herceptin®), ramucirumab (Cyramza™)
Systemic mastocytosis	Imatinib mesylate (Gleevec®)
Thyroid cancer	Cabozantinib (Cometriq™), vandetanib (Caprelsa®), sorafenib (Nexavar®)

[a] An updated list can be found at the NCI website: http://www.cancer.gov/about-cancer/treatment/types/targeted-therapies/targeted-therapies-fact-sheet.

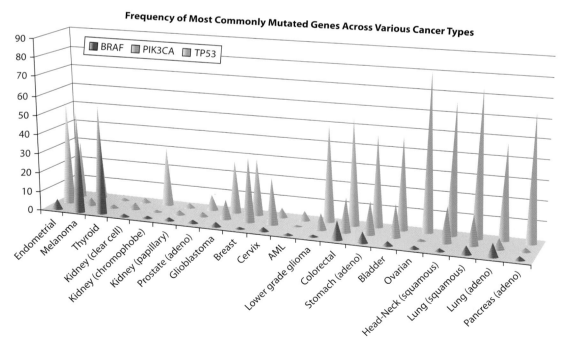

Figure 9-2. Frequency of the most commonly mutated genes (*BRAF, PIK3CA,* and *TP53*) across various cancer types. (Data from Martincorena I, Campbell PJ: Somatic mutation in cancer and normal cells, *Science*. 2015 Sep 25;349(6255):1483-1489).

the premise that a treatment that works against a mutated target in one cancer may in theory work against that same target in a different cancer. While there are several examples of successful off-label use of targeted cancer treatment in different cancers[6-8], evidence suggests that this is not always the case. For example, the drug vemurafenib was developed to treat *BRAF*-mutated melanoma. *BRAF* is mutated in other tumor types as well, such as colorectal cancer, but treatment of these other *BRAF*-mutated tumors with vemurafenib resulted in successful treatment of some, but not all of the tumor types[9].

A number of basket trials, such as the one testing vemurafenib across different *BRAF*-mutated cancer types, are currently underway to test the efficacy of therapies against a specific molecular target independent of histology[10].

In addition to FDA-approved therapies, there are numerous targeted therapies in various stages of clinical development, catalogued in the U.S. National Cancer Institute clinical trials database (www.clinicaltrials.gov). Knowledge of a patient's tumor profile could inform eligibility for one of these trials.

Non-small cell lung carcinoma exemplifies the diversity in major cancer drivers found among different patients and the large armamentarium of treatment options available. Three FDA-approved treatments directed against two molecular targets, EGFR and ALK, are available for NSCLC patients. A number of additional targets frequently found in NSCLC patients (BRAF, DDR2, HER2, MEK1, RET) have FDA-approved drugs in other cancer types and could be used off-label. Finally, there are clinical trials available for at least two additional targets found in NSCLC patients, AKT1 and KRAS. Overall, 75% of NSCLC patients have treatment options, with over half of these for FDA-approved treatments.

Several cancers have targeted treatment options for the majority of patients (Fig. 9-3)[11]. Most patients with melanoma or colorectal cancer will have a mutation in their tumor that is amenable to targeted treatment. There are other cancers, such as head and neck or neuroendocrine system cancers, where there are fewer patients with known viable targeted treatment options based on their tumor profile.

> **Key Point**
>
> Tumor profiling has been shown to be clinically useful in cases where there is no standard of care or when the standard of care has been exhausted, including the following situations:
>
> - In patients with rare cancers
> - In patients with refractory disease who have failed first- or second-line therapy
> - In patients with advanced, or aggressive cancer

INDICATIONS FOR USE OF TUMOR PROFILING FOR EXPANDED TREATMENT OPTIONS

Tumor profiling is currently not used on newly diagnosed cancers when a standard of care treatment is available. However, in time as more evidence is accumulated, it is expected to become part of routine standard of care.

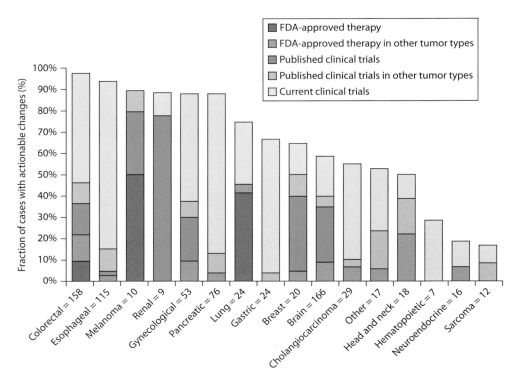

Figure 9-3. Clinically actionable somatic genomic alterations in various tumor types (Reproduced with permission from Jones S, Anagnostou V, Lytle K, et al: Personalized genomic analyses for cancer mutation discovery and interpretation, *Sci Transl Med.* 2015 Apr 15;7(283):283ra53).

Each bar represents the fraction of cases with mutations in clinically actionable genes as determined by the comparison of alterations to genes that were associated with established FDA-approved therapies (brown), previously published clinical trials (green), or current clinical trials in the same tumor type (blue). For approved therapies and previously published clinical trials, potential actionability was also considered in tumor types that were different from those where the clinical use has been described (light brown and light green, respectively). Some of the colorectal tumors analyzed were from patients with tumors known to be *KRAS* wild type, resulting in a lower fraction of cases with actionable changes related to FDA-approved therapies.

SELECTING A LABORATORY AND TUMOR PROFILING TEST FOR EXPANDED TREATMENT OPTIONS

There are dozens of laboratories that offer tumor profiling for cancer treatment. The laboratories with the most experience in the United States include those listed in Table 9-3.

All of these laboratories offer tumor profiling for solid tumors, including analysis of multiple genes, or gene panels. Most target specific hotspots (regions of the gene where known mutations tend to cluster) in a defined set of

Table 9-3. List of U.S. laboratories with extensive experience using molecular tumor profiling

Laboratory	Link
Caris Diagnostics	http://www.carislifesciences.com/
Foundation Medicine	https://www.foundationmedicine.com/
Paradigm	http://www.paradigmdx.org/
Personal Genome Diagnostics	http://www.personalgenome.com/
Several major U.S. medical centers	—

genes, while others offer more comprehensive sequencing of the entire gene region. Besides gene sequencing for detecting DNA variation, labs also offer immunohistochemical, RNA expression, and/or a variety of post-translational modification analyses. A subset will offer tumor profiling for hematological malignancies. The main considerations when choosing a laboratory for tumor profiling include the following.

Types of variants detected

Tumor profiling should detect a wide range of relevant DNA alterations:

- Single nucleotide variants (SNVs)
- Small insertions/deletions (InDels)
- Copy number changes (CNVs), including amplification or deletion of the entire gene
- Structural variants (SVs), including inversions and translocations that result in fusion genes

Other relevant alterations in a tumor include differences in gene or protein expression, often the result of epigenetic modification to the DNA.

Complementary methods may be required to capture all of the relevant somatic variations in a tumor. Panel-based next-generation sequencing is a cost-effective means of capturing variation due to DNA alterations (SNVs, InDels, CNVs, SVs) in a subset of genes and gene regions. Some laboratories opt for more robust technologies like fluorescence in situ hybridization (FISH) to capture some of the larger DNA alterations. Immunohistochemistry (IHC) and mRNA expression are both suitable for capturing alterations in gene expression.

Sequence coverage

Next-generation sequencing panels are designed to have excellent *breadth* of coverage of the gene regions on the panel. *Depth* of coverage is a metric that reflects the sensitivity of variant detection. In germline sequencing, an average depth of coverage of about 30× is sufficient for detecting variation, because the sample is homogeneous, but since tumor biopsy specimens are complex mixtures of heterogeneous subclones of the tumor, as well as surrounding normal tissue, higher coverage is needed for accurate somatic variant detection. To detect a variant present in 5% or more of the tissue sample, a minimum coverage of 400–500× is required, and the sample must consist of at least about 20% tumor, as determined by a pathology exam. Coverage above 500× may be able to detect minor variations, found in a small percentage of tumor cells, but this variation may be less relevant and at the expense of increased tissue requirement and cost.

Tumor versus normal

The presence of acquired (somatic) DNA alterations is sometimes assessed by comparing tumor DNA to normal, nontumor DNA from the same individual. In this case, sample requirements for tumor profiling include not just the tumor sample, but either blood, saliva, or buccal swab specimens as well (note: sequencing the matched normal DNA may not be covered by insurance, even if the tumor gene panel is). Sequencing normal DNA and then subtracting out the germline variation can quantitatively verify somatic variation. However, not all laboratories use normal DNA subtraction. Instead, most use statistical approaches to subtract out variation known to be present in the general (healthy) population. While not as accurate as sequencing and subtracting out matched normal DNA variants, this approach is valid for targeted analysis of small gene panels that assess well-studied regions of the genome. Jones et al[11]. published an analysis of tumor alone versus tumor-normal methods for detecting somatic variation in large gene panels and exome sequencing. They found that failure to subtract out matched normal DNA could lead to detection of germline variants that would be erroneously classified as somatic in some cases, resulting in inappropriate direction of therapy.

Laboratories that perform tumor-normal analyses (and even those that do tumor-only testing) have the capability to identify germline cancer predisposing alleles in patients. Jones et al[11] found such pathogenic or likely pathogenic mutations in 3% of their adult cancer patients, while a recent study of pediatric cancers found 8.5% of children and adolescents harbored a germline cancer predisposing allele[12]. This has implications for family members of the patient, who may seek testing for these variants to assess their own risk of developing cancer. The probability of finding predisposition mutations depends highly on the genes analyzed in the first place, and is less likely in the case of small gene panels.

Number of genes

The number of genes analyzed in a tumor profiling test varies by laboratory. In fact, laboratories may only query gene hotspots, locations in the gene where the most common variants are found. As with hereditary cancer predisposition panels, analyzing more genes is not always better. Smaller panels of genes may only include those genes that direct use of an FDA-approved drug. Larger gene panels may include those genes in the pathway of certain cancers, or otherwise related to cancer, with no FDA-approved therapies, but possible investigational therapies available. Whole-genome/exome analysis with or without additional gene expression analysis represents the broadest survey of genetic aberrations. As the number of genes grows, it's increasingly likely that more actionable changes will be identified. However, it comes at a cost of more uncertainty as more variants of uncertain significance will be identified.

Turnaround time

Although most commercial laboratories quote turnaround times of less than two weeks, academic labs tend to take longer. The experience of at least one academic medical center was a median of 27 days from the time the tests were ordered until results were available[13]. However, this included a median of 11 days required for the tissue specimen to be obtained and sent to the laboratory.

Invasiveness

Liquid biopsies that capture circulating tumor DNA offer an alternative to invasive tumor tissue biopsies used for tumor profiling to help match patients to drugs. This technology has already been used to detect residual disease and to monitor relapse using samples of blood or even urine, but is now beginning to branch into the area of identifying associated treatment options. Several companies offer blood-based tests for treatment matching, using either analysis of gene hotspots or broader gene sequencing panels (e.g., Guardant Health).

SPECIMEN REQUIREMENTS

Laboratories have slightly different sample requirements for performing tumor profiling. In general, labs require formalin-fixed, paraffin-embedded (FFPE) tumor specimens of a certain volume, comprised of at least 20% tumor tissue. Unstained slides can also be used for profiling and are sometimes required for IHC. See company websites for more details on sample requirements.

LIMITATIONS OF TUMOR PROFILING

As tumors grow, they continue to acquire mutations and evolve through clonal expansion and selection. The result is that a tumor is heterogeneous, comprised of different subclones spatially separated or intermingled through-out the tumor (Fig. 9-4)[14]. Intratumor heterogeneity has implications for tumor profiling. A single biopsy specimen may not be representative of all of the relevant subclones of the tumor. It is estimated that only about 30% of the somatic mutations detected in the primary tumor are ubiquitous[15]. When repeat testing is required, a new biopsy is desirable, especially after treatment, as the predominant subclones may have changed.

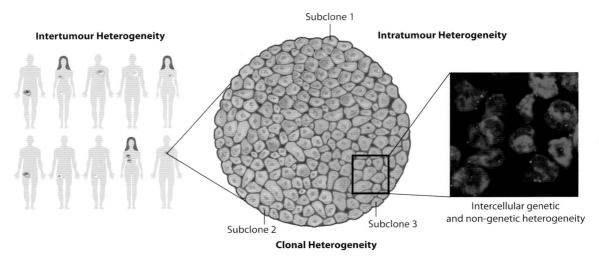

Figure 9-4. Intertumour and intratumour heterogeneity (Reproduced with permission from Burrell RA, McGranahan N, Bartek J, et al: The causes and consequences of genetic heterogeneity in cancer evolution, *Nature.* 2013 Sep 19;501(7467):338-345).

Genetic and phenotypic variations are observed between tumors of different tissue and cell types, as well as between individuals with the same tumour type (intertumor heterogeneity). Within a tumour, subclonal diversity may be observed (intratumour heterogeneity). Subclones may intermingle (as shown by subclones 1 and 2) or be spatially separated (as shown by subclone 3). Separation between subclones could reflect physical barriers such as blood vessels or microenvironmental changes. Tumor subclones may show differential gene expression due to both genetic and epigenetic heterogeneity. Within a subclonal population of tumor cells—shown here as a tumor section, hybridized to two fluorescent probes for the centromeres of two chromosomes (chromosome 2, red; chromosome 18, green) with DNA (blue) there is intercellular genetic and nongenetic variation of, for example, chromosome copy number, somatic point mutations, or epigenetic modifications that results in phenotypic diversity. Intercellular genetic heterogeneity is exacerbated by genomic instability, and may foster the emergence of tumor subclones. Genomic instability and tumor subclonal architecture may vary further over time if influenced by, for example, cancer treatment.

Tumors are under selective pressure and it is not uncommon for a targeted treatment to be effective initially, only to have the patient develop resistance. Resistance usually results from expansion of minor subclones, unaffected by the targeted treatment, with different driver mutations. This has led some to consider combination therapy for cancer[16].

GUIDELINES FOR USE OF TUMOR PROFILING PANELS TO DIRECT TREATMENT

The analytical validity, clinical validity, and clinical utility of using tumor profiling panels to direct treatment was assessed in a 2014 report from PLoS Currents Evidence on Genomic Tests[17]. They found a dearth of evidence supporting clinical validity for most genes on large gene panels. Even for genes that demonstrate clinical validity for directing treatment in cancer, evidence for using that same gene to guide treatment in another cancer (off-label use) is typically not available. With regard to clinical utility, they report the following:

- No evidence of improved treatment outcomes from using large gene panels to direct therapy in solid tumors.

- A potential harm related to incidental findings that the test providers are not equipped to handle.

- Another potential harm related to uncertainty in the cost-benefit ratio of the off-label use of expensive chemotherapeutic drugs with well-characterized adverse effects.

In contrast, the Center for Medical Technology Policy drafted somewhat more optimistic guidelines[3]:

- Recognition that evidence of clinical validity for every gene on a panel may not currently be available, but that panels with at least five genes supported by evidence should be covered.

- Recognition that clinical utility is limited, but that benefits in terms of survival and quality of life may outweigh the risks in certain populations where standard of care has failed or does not exist.

INTERPRETING TUMOR PROFILING REPORTS FOR EXPANDED TREATMENT OPTIONS

Despite the high mutational burden of tumors (average of 33–66 mutated genes per tumor), laboratory reports from targeted tumor profiling usually contain an average of only 2–4 variants (due to the limited number of genes and gene hotspots tested)[11]. A typical laboratory report will include actionable findings, that is, a known pathogenic variant in a known gene target or prognostic marker for an FDA-approved or investigational drug. The report may include other relevant variants in oncogenes or tumor suppressors that are not immediately actionable, but may be informative. The report may also include variants of uncertain significance, where the pathogenicity of the variant is in question, or where variants in the gene are not convincingly linked to treatment outcome.

To fully appreciate the results in a tumor profiling report, it is helpful to understand how the results are generated. When a tumor is analyzed for the presence of mutations in panel genes, many variants may be found, but not all will impact the efficacy of the drug. It is the job of the qualified laboratory personnel to determine the following:

---

[3] CMTP. Initial Medical Policy and Model Coverage Guidelines for Clinical Next Generation Sequencing in Oncology Report and Recommendations. Retrieved from Green Park Collaborative of the Center for Medical Technology. 2015. Available at: http://www.cmtpnet.org/docs/resources/Full_Re lease_Version_August_13

Is the mutation real?

A series of quality control filters, including things like sequencing coverage, are typically applied to the data to ensure that the mutation is real and not an artifact.

Does the variant alter the function of the protein?

Variants are evaluated for allele frequency, presence in variant databases, functional prediction algorithms, and other computational tools to determine the likelihood of altering the protein function.

Is the gene actionable?

A body of evidence linking the molecular alteration to treatment options is reviewed. Laboratories curate information from drug-gene databases, knowledge bases, the scientific literature, and clinical trials resources. The evidence supporting an assertion is a key element to the report, allowing the provider to independently judge the relevance of the findings in the context of their patient. The evidence may be curated from only human clinical trials or may expand to basic science literature. Differences in the level of evidence are taken into account, when determining treatment.

The depth of these curation efforts, as well as experience, can distinguish one lab's interpretation and reporting from the next. There is no standardization in interpretation and reporting, although some groups have recently proposed a standard classification systems for somatic variants detected via molecular profiling[19,20].

Some institutions invoke the help of molecular tumor boards to facilitate further interpretation of tumor profiling reports and to propose treatment strategies[21]. In addition to clinical professionals, molecular tumor boards also may enlist the expertise of basic scientists, geneticists, and bioinformaticians.

MANAGING EXPECTATIONS

In practice, a survey of the National Comprehensive Cancer Network (NCCN) member institutions using tumor profiling found that for most institutions (82%), even though tumors were found to have actionable mutations, the results of tumor profiling influenced the care of less than half of the patients tested[22]. This speaks largely to the challenges of enrolling patients in clinical trials, including strict eligibility criteria and geographical hurdles, as well as access to drugs.

POTENTIAL FOR GERMLINE FINDINGS IN TUMOR SEQUENCING

Germline variants can be identified and/or inferred from tumor sequencing results, even without direct analysis of germline DNA[11]. Routine clinical tumor profiling in one study revealed that 13% of patients carried a germline mutation in a cancer susceptibility gene[23]. Presence of a potentially pathogenic somatic variant in a gene known to underlie inherited cancer may turn out to be germline and should be followed up.

Practice Point: Clinical Scenario 1

A patient had their tumor profiled to determine the best course of treatment and in the process was found to carry a germline cancer variant in TP53, a high risk gene for Li–Fraumeni syndrome. How should one proceed?

If the variant is found using an assay that examined tumor only, the first step is to obtain a germline DNA sample (from blood, saliva, buccal swab, for example) and verify that it is indeed germline. The laboratory that performed the tumor profiling may offer confirmatory testing themselves or in partnership with a reference lab. Confirmatory testing may or may not be covered by insurance.

   If confirmed, it is recommended that the patient be referred to a genetic counselor or other genetics professional, who can help clarify risks associated with an inherited cancer predisposition for themselves and their family and assist in establishing an appropriate screening regimen for future cancers. Occasionally, knowledge of germline variants may alter the course of treatment for the patient. Genetic counselors can facilitate communication of results with other family members of the patient. For more information see Raymond et al[24].

Practice Point: Clinical Scenario 2

A patient had their tumor profiled to determine the best course of treatment and the report indicates multiple actionable genomic alterations. The alterations include two targetable changes, both for drugs in early phase clinical development. How should one proceed?

Tumor profiling reports should provide a summary of the evidence supporting each genetic alteration and the treatment recommendations. This evidence will need to be reviewed by the treating physician to determine the most viable strategy. Consideration should be given to not only the strength of evidence supporting the recommended treatment option, but the likelihood of obtaining that treatment. Often the best option is to discuss these findings with a molecular tumor board.

RESOURCES

My Cancer Genome (http://www.mycancergenome.org/)

From the Vanderbilt-Ingram Cancer Center, My Cancer Genome is a personalized cancer medicine knowledge resource that gives up-to-date information on what mutations make cancers grow and related therapeutic implications, including available clinical trials.

Clinical trials (www.Clinicaltrials.gov)

ClinicalTrials.gov is a web-based resource that provides users with easy access to information on publicly and privately supported clinical studies on a wide range of diseases and conditions.

ASCO University Molecular Oncology Tumor Boards (http://university .asco.org/motb)

The Molecular Oncology Tumor Boards are a series of monthly user-driven discussions designed to help cancer care providers with the interpretation and understanding of tumor molecular profiling tests and studies.

CSER consortium (www.cser-consortium.org)

The National Human Genome Research Institute/National Cancer Institute—supported Clinical Sequencing Exploratory Research (CSER) Consortium—includes three sites serving both pediatric and adult oncology patient populations that are studying the implementation of genomics in clinical oncology and returning genomic results to oncologists and patients.

REFERENCES

1. Vogelstein B, Papadopoulos N, Velculescu VE, Zhou S, Diaz LA Jr, Kinzler KW. Cancer genome landscapes. *Science*. 2013;339:1546-1558.
2. Alexandrov LB, Nik-Zainal S, Wedge DC, et al. Signatures of mutational processes in human cancer. *Nature*. 2013;500:415-421.
3. Garraway LA. Genomics-driven oncology: framework for an emerging paradigm. *J Clin Oncol*. 2013;31:1806-1814.
4. Sestak I, Cuzick J. Markers for the identification of late breast cancer recurrence. *Breast Cancer Res*. 2015;17:10.
5. Martincorena I, Campbell PJ. Somatic mutation in cancer and normal cells. *Science*. 2015;349:1483-1489.
6. Iyer G, Hanrahan AJ, Milowsky MI, et al. Genome sequencing identifies a basis for everolimus sensitivity. *Science*. 2012; 338:221.
7. Sen B, Peng S, Tang X, et al. Kinase-impaired BRAF mutations in lung cancer confer sensitivity to dasatinib. *Sci Transl Med*. 2012;4:136ra170.
8. Serra V, Vivancos A, Puente XS, et al. Clinical response to a lapatinib-based therapy for a Li-Fraumeni syndrome patient with a novel HER2V659E mutation. *Cancer Discov*. 2013;3:1238-1244.
9. Hyman DM, Puzanov I, Subbiah V, et al. Vemurafenib in multiple nonmelanoma cancers with BRAF V600 mutations. *N Engl J Med*. 2015;373:726-736.
10. Redig AJ, Janne PA. Basket trials and the evolution of clinical trial design in an era of genomic medicine. *J Clin Oncol*. 2015;33:975-977.
11. Jones S, Anagnostou V, Lytle K, et al. Personalized genomic analyses for cancer mutation discovery and interpretation. *Sci Transl Med*. 2015;7:283ra253.
12. Zhang J, Walsh MF, Wu G, et al. Germline mutations in predisposition genes in pediatric cancer. *N Engl J Med*. 2015;373:2336-2346.

13. Schwaederle M, Parker BA, Schwab RB, et al. Molecular tumor board: the University of California-San Diego Moores Cancer Center experience. *Oncologist*. 2014;19:631-636.
14. Burrell RA, McGranahan N, Bartek J, Swanton C. The causes and consequences of genetic heterogeneity in cancer evolution. *Nature*. 2013;501:338-345.
15. Gerlinger M, Rowan AJ, Horswell S, et al. Intratumor heterogeneity and branched evolution revealed by multiregion sequencing. *N Engl J Med*. 2012;366:883-892.
16. Al-Lazikani B, Banerji U, Workman P. Combinatorial drug therapy for cancer in the post-genomic era. *Nat Biotechnol*. 2012;30:679-692.
17. Marrone M, Filipski KK, Gillanders EM, Schully SD, Freedman AN. Multi-marker solid tumor panels using next-generation sequencing to direct molecularly targeted therapies. *PLoS Curr*. 2014;6.
18. Sukhai MA, Craddock KJ, Thomas M, et al. A classification system for clinical relevance of somatic variants identified in molecular profiling of cancer. *Genet Med*. 2015.
19. Van Allen EM, Wagle N, Stojanov P, et al. Whole-exome sequencing and clinical interpretation of formalin-fixed, paraffin-embedded tumor samples to guide precision cancer medicine. *Nat Med*. 2014;20:682-688.
20. Erdmann J. All aboard: will molecular tumor boards help cancer patients? *Nat Med*. 2015;21:655-656.
21. Kurzrock R, Colevas AD, Olszanski A, et al. NCCN Oncology Research Program's Investigator Steering Committee and NCCN Best Practices Committee Molecular Profiling Surveys. *J Natl Compr Canc Netw*. 2015;13:1337-1346.
22. Schrader KA, Cheng DT, Joseph V, et al. Germline variants in targeted tumor sequencing using matched normal DNA. *JAMA Oncol*. 2015;1-8.
23. Raymond VM, Gray SW, Roychowdhury S, et al. Germline findings in tumor-only sequencing: points to consider for clinicians and laboratories. *J Natl Cancer Inst*. 2016;108.

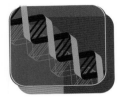

CHAPTER 10

The Brain

Clinical applications in the area of neurology, neurodegeneration, and psychiatric disease are still limited to the diagnosis of rare or early-onset disorders and using pharmacogenomic markers to predict efficacy of treatments. Research aimed at using genomics to predict idiopathic causes of dementia, movement disorders, and many psychiatric conditions is one of the hottest fields in medicine and undoubtedly this chapter will be considerably longer in future editions. A few areas are worthy of consideration here.

GENETIC TESTING FOR HEREDITARY ALZHEIMER AND PARKINSON DISEASE

It has been recognized for decades that neurodegenerative disorders can occur in families, in a dominant or recessive fashion, and identifying the genetic underpinnings has been pivotal in the current understanding of the pathophysiology of these disorders. There is clearly much in common between rare heritable forms of neurodegenerative disease and the more common so-called idiopathic or late-onset disease. A discussion of each single-gene disorder is beyond the scope of this text, but what has changed in the genomics era is the discovery of many more Mendelian causes of a variety of dementia, movement disorders, ataxia, and other neurodegenerative diseases. Thanks to whole-exome sequencing, identifying causative mutations in early-onset neurodegeneration families has been greatly accelerated, and even single individuals with atypical neurodegeneration can sometimes yield novel genetic insight.

At this time, absent a family history, there are no formal recommendations for screening healthy individuals for early-onset neurodegenerative disease. The clearly monogenic forms of these conditions are sufficiently rare, and too few treatments are available, that broad screening would not be cost-effective or likely to provide actionable information. Nevertheless, as sequencing becomes less expensive and is available direct-to-consumer, screening for early-onset neurodegeneration is likely to occur indirectly and must be dealt with thoughtfully. Neurodegeneration is particularly challenging from a screening standpoint because individuals in the same family with the same mutation can have very different ages of onset and severity of disease. Further, the prospect of loss of cognitive or motor function can be the most disturbing to a person of any possible health outcome.

For patients with early-onset dementia or movement disorders, investigation for monogenic causes is appropriate and should start with a detailed family history. Often a neurologist rather than a geneticist will undertake this evaluation and many neurologists specialize in dementia and movement disorders. Single gene and panel testing is available for known Alzheimer and Parkinson genes, though new genes are being discovered all the time (refer to Appendix 5 for guidance finding and selecting available tests).

APOE TESTING FOR PREDISPOSITION TO ALZHEIMER DISEASE

One particular neurodegeneration risk factor bears special mention. The E4 allele of apolipoprotein E (ApoE4) certainly confers an increased lifetime risk of developing Alzheimer disease, and at a younger age than individuals without this allele. Persons carrying one copy have a 1.5 to twofold increased odds of developing Alzheimer disease while those carrying two copies of the E4 allele are at four- to tenfold increased odds. The effect of the variant also differs by race and gender. This strong association has led to the consideration of this allele as a useful diagnostic and prognostic marker for Alzheimer disease. It is neither! An ApoE4 allele is neither sufficient nor necessary to cause Alzheimer disease. The American College of Medical Genetics and Genomics (ACMG), as part of the American Board of Internal Medicine Foundation's Choosing Wisely® program, has clearly stated that testing for ApoE4 status is almost never indicated in assessing the risk, diagnosis, prognosis, or treatment of Alzheimer disease. Testing for this allele is widely available, including as part of large gene panels for much more penetrant risk factors for Alzheimer. Hopefully, with ongoing research, other genetic and environmental risk factors might be combined with ApoE4 status to provide a more accurate and clinically meaningful assessment.

GENETIC TESTING FOR PSYCHIATRIC DISEASE

To date, the major contributions of genomic medicine to psychiatric disease have been in the research arena, but translation to diagnostics and therapeutics is unquestionably certain to follow. Like research in autism (see Chapter 5), studies of disorders such as bipolar and schizophrenia are uncovering the role for rare and de novo mutations in these conditions, and are highlighting critical neurodevelopmental processes that contribute to their onset and symptomatology.

One aspect already benefiting from genomic technology is the ability to detect forms of mental illness that are caused by known biochemical disorders. These associations have been recognized for years, but the increasing ease of testing for many conditions simultaneously is starting to improve diagnostic rates. Metabolic syndromes that can present primarily or exclusively as psychiatric disease include Niemann–Pick type C, Wilson Disease, phenylketonuria (PKU), porphyrias, cerebrotendinous xanthomatosis, homocystinurias, defects in cobalamin processing, and some urea cycle disorders[1]. Many chromosomal microdeletion syndromes also predispose to psychiatric disease. The list of all Mendelian disorders that could possibly present psychiatrically is much longer, and certainly more remain to be discovered. Some percentage of institutionalized or incarcerated individuals probably has one of these diagnoses. Critically, some of these disorders can be treated or managed, thus making a diagnosis vastly preferable to nonspecific psychoactive medications.

From a societal standpoint, we tend to view antisocial behavior differently when it occurs in the context of a genetic diagnosis, and thus we owe it to individuals to provide appropriate testing when indicated. Unfortunately, the mentally ill are most at risk for being un- or underinsured, and thus access to genomic technologies lags for this population. Further, gene panels for single-gene causes of mental illness (particularly psychosis) are lacking, and numerous metabolic tests would need to be sent to cover all possible diagnoses.

PHARMACOGENOMIC TESTS FOR SELECTING TREATMENTS FOR PSYCHIATRIC DISORDERS

The psychiatric drugs listed in Table 10-1 contain information in the U.S. Food and Drug Administration (FDA) label relating to pharmacogenomic testing, however none of these meet the U.S. Centers for Disease Control and Prevention (CDC) Tier 1 level of evidence sufficiently enough to support implementation into practice. They are all CDC Tier 2, with insufficient evidence yet potentially useful for informing selective use strategies. There are no professional guidelines for recommending when to order one of these tests. If genotype information is already available on the patient, Clinical Pharmacogenomics Implementation Consortium (CPIC) guidelines, when available, can be used to interpret genotypes and guide treatment decisions.

Despite the Tier 2 ranking of these tests, several laboratories offer neuropsychiatric pharmacogenetic panels to guide antidepressant and antipsychotic treatment selection (e.g., companies AssureRx, Genelex, Genomind, Pathway Genomics, Molecular diagnostics lab, Progenity, and others) and health care providers are using these tests.

According to the CDC tiered assessment, currently there is insufficient evidence to support pharmacogenomic testing of Cytochrome P450 (CYP) genes for improving the efficacy of selective serotonin reuptake inhibitors (SSRIs) in nonpsychotic depression (http://www.egappreviews.org/recommendations/depression.htm).

Table 10-1. CDC Tier 2 pharmacogenomic tests for treating psychiatric disorders.

Drug	Indication	Gene(s)	CPIC
Amitriptyline	Depression	CYP2D6	2013
Desipramine	Depression	CYP2D6	2013
Imipramine	Depression	CYP2D6	2013
Nortriptyline	Depression	CYP2D6	2013
Trimipramine	Depression	CYP2D6	2013
Citalopram	Depression	CYP2C19, CYP2D6	
Doxepin	Insomnia	CYP2D6, CYP2C19	2013
Fluvoxamine	Obsessive-compulsive disorder	CYP2D6, CYP2C19	
Clomipramine	Obsessive-compulsive disorder	CYP2D6	2013
Atomoxetine	Attention-deficit/hyperactivity disorder	CYP2D6	
Fluoxetine	Major depressive disorder, obsessive-compulsive disorder, bulimia nervosa, panic disorder	CYP2D6	
Venlafaxine	Major depressive disorder, social anxiety disorder	CYP2D6	
Modafinil	Narcolepsy, obstructive sleep apnea, and shift work disorder	CYP2D6	
Iloperidone	Schizophrenia	CYP2D6	
Risperidone	Schizophrenia, bipolar I disorder, autistic disorder	CYP2D6	
Aripiprazole	Schizophrenia, bipolar I disorder, major depressive disorder, autistic disorder	CYP2D6	
Clozapine	Schizophrenia, schizoaffective disorder	CYP2D6	

CPIC, Clinical Pharmacogenomics Implementation Consortium, refers to guidelines for using pharmacogenomic information to guide treatment in patients.

Providers interested in offering pharmacogenomic tests to their psychiatric patients should review summaries and evidence found on the PharmGKB website (pharmgkb.org). Information about ordering tests can be found in Appendix 5. Additional pharmacogenomic resources can be found in Chapter 6.

Practice Point: Clinical Scenario

A patient presents to you with depression. Before you initiate treatment with citalopram, the patient gives you the results from a direct-to-consumer genetic testing (a test they were able to order themselves) of their CYP2C19 gene, which showed that they are a poor metabolizer (CYP2C19*2/*2). CPIC guidelines recommend reducing the dose of the drug in your patient. How do you use this information to make a treatment decision?

Consider the following:

1. Is an alternative treatment available that has similar efficacy to citalopram and is not affected by these gene variants? If so, you may choose to use that drug.
2. How will poor metabolism affect drug concentration? In this case, poor metabolizers may accumulate drug in their body, increasing their risk of side effects.
3. What are the side effects? Are they severe? Does their risk outweigh the risk of underdosing and possibly compromising the efficacy of the drug for treating depression?
4. If the patient was already taking the medication with a clinical response and no side effects, would you change the dose based on these results?

RESOURCES

National Coalition for Health Professional Education in Genetics (http://www.nchpeg.org/index.php?option=com_content&view=article&id=118&Item id=118)

An introduction to psychiatric genetics for genetic counselors with additional helpful links.

Alzheimer's Association (http://www.alz.org/alzheimers_disease_1973.asp)

A large advocacy, research, and education group for patients, families, caregivers, and professionals who interact with Alzheimer disease. Also contains information about genetics and risk factors.

The Michael J. Fox Foundation (https://www.michaeljfox.org/)

A large foundation dedicated to understanding and treating Parkinson disease, which includes links ("Understanding Parkinson's") and discussion about the genetics and promising research in the field.

REFERENCE

1. Klunemann HH, Santosh PJ, Sedel F. Treatable metabolic psychoses that go undetected: what Niemann-Pick type C can teach us. *Int J Psychiatry Clin Pract.* 2012;16(3):162-169. doi:10.3109/13651501.2012.687451.

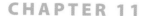

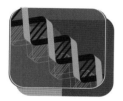

CHAPTER 11

Wellness

Over a million people have taken advantage of direct-to-consumer genetic testing, mostly through the genetic testing company 23andMe. Some are motivated by the desire to know their ancestry, while others hope to gain insight into their disease risks. We are also seeing the launch of dozens of local and international projects that will generate, and hopefully return results of the genome sequences of millions of people. These include efforts by the U.S. Precision Medicine Initiative Cohort, Human Longevity, Inc., the Million Vets Program, Genome England's 100K Genome Project, the Saudi Human Genome Program, and others[1]. It is expected that genome sequencing will become a part of routine health care in the not too distant future. Most of this sequencing will be done on ostensibly healthy individuals. Health care providers need to be aware of the value and limitations of genome sequencing, as they will likely encounter a patient who has this information in hand and asks them what it means. This chapter will help prepare health care providers for a healthy patient coming to them with their genomic information.

WHOLE GENOME/EXOME SEQUENCING VERSUS TARGETED GENOTYPING

Many people who have had their genomes analyzed on the 23andMe targeted genotyping platform think they've had their whole genome sequenced. While they indeed have had many of their variants analyzed, there is a distinction. Figure 11-1 illustrates the difference in the number of nucleotide positions querried by whole genome sequencing, whole exome sequencing, and 23andMe. Both whole-genome sequencing (WGS) and whole-exome sequencing (WES) are designed to detect any of the variants that a person's genome may contain either in their whole genome or only in their exome. In contrast, 23andMe uses a targeted genotyping method where the variants that can be detected have been selected a priori. They include mostly variants in the noncoding (nonexome) region of the genome, along with a select set of exome variants, chosen for their role in disease.

> ### Key Point
>
> Both WGS and WES have known gaps in their coverage of certain difficult to sequence gene regions, some of which harbor important disease genes, so in fact "whole" genomes and exomes are not entirely complete with current technology. One study reported that, among 56 important high-risk disease genes, about 10–20% were not adequately covered by WGS[2]. In the diagnostic setting, laboratories often employ enrichment strategies to panels of very important genes to improve the quality of the data. Standard WGS and WES do not employ these tactics.

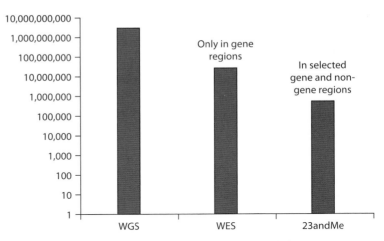

Figure 11-1. Comparison of nucleotide positions queried by whole-genome sequencing (WGS), whole-exome sequencing (WES), and 23andMe.

WHAT CAN OSTENSIBLY HEALTHY INDIVIDUALS LEARN FROM THEIR GENOME?

The ability to glean health information from a genome is determined in part by the platform used to detect the genetic variants and in part by the interpretation and annotation of the variants identified. Both aspects are addressed below, where we provide a general ranking of each platform (gold, silver, bronze).

Whole-genome sequencing

Gold level—in terms of the breadth of clinically relevant variation that can be detected. This platform is capable of detecting most Mendelian dominant, Mendelian recessive, pharmacogenes, and common disease variants. The reason for saying most and not all is because some of the types of disease-causing variants (e.g., trinucleotide repeats) are not detected well, nor are variants in genes that have high homology with other genes (unfortunately this includes important pharmacogenes like *CYP2D6* and the human leukocyte antigen (HLA) genes).

WGS is currently expensive (hovering around $1000 for the sequencing alone) and the results that are returned depend on where the sequencing is done. At the moment there are not many options for obtaining clinical-grade WGS along with interpretation, but the landscape is rapidly changing. WGS is the gift that keeps on giving. A person can have their genome sequenced once, and interpreted for many years to come. Also, technological advances are permitting more difficult regions of the genome to be sequenced and WGS should move closer to fully deserving its moniker *whole* genome.

Whole-exome sequencing

Silver level—the sequencing technology only captures variation in the coding region of the genome (about 1.5% of the genome), but it is this region that harbors the majority of variations underlying Mendelian diseases (dominant and recessive), as well as about 70% of important pharmacogenomic variants[3]. It has the advantage over WGS of being less expensive to generate the sequence data, but much of the cost for both WGS and WES is in the interpretation of variants.

In terms of variants underlying common, complex diseases, there are a few such as specific variants of *APOE* for Alzheimer disease, the Factor V Leiden variant for deep vein thrombosis, and others that WES can detect, which might provide desired information to individuals to manage their risk. But, the majority of variants for complex diseases, as well as about 30% of pharmacogenomic variants, are not in the exome and will be missed by WES. For example, warfarin sensitivity is determined by two coding-region variants in *CYP2C9*, but also a promoter region variant in *VKORC1*, the latter of which would not be detected by WES.

23andMe

Bronze level—in terms of the breadth of variants detected, but it has some advantages over the other platforms. At a price point of <$200, it is the most economical means of obtaining a large amount of genetic information. Their targeted genotyping platform captures recognized pharmacogenomic variants in the exome and noncoding region of the genome, and common disease variants as well. The drawback of 23andMe is that for Mendelian diseases, their platform captures only a small subset of the known pathogenic variants for selected diseases. For example, over 1000 pathogenic variants have been described in each of the inherited breast cancer genes, *BRCA1* and *BRCA2*, and yet 23andMe only tests for three of them. Similarly, there are over 500 known pathogenic variants (and probably many more exceedingly rare ones yet to be discovered) in the cystic fibrosis gene, *CFTR*, and yet 23andMe only tests for 26 of the most common ones. Practically, an individual who tested negative by the 23andMe *CFTR* variant panel would have a higher residual risk of actually being a cystic fibrosis carrier than someone who underwent sequencing of the entire gene (though residual risk never gets to zero). Thus, for example, for the partner of a known CF carrier, targeted mutation testing would not be the preferred test (see Chapter 1).

Another aspect of 23andMe worth mentioning is the interpretation of variants. Prior to being asked by the FDA to cease delivering health information to consumers, the evidence curation, interpretation, and explanation of results for individual variants offered by 23andMe was of very high quality. Level of evidence supporting genetic associations was graded with a number of stars to indicate confidence of each result. Risk estimates were generated from large studies. Where relevant, the limitations of testing a subset of known variants for Mendelian diseases were pointed out. Where they got into trouble was primarily in the area of common, complex diseases (health risks) where individual variants with little predictive value were combined into polygenic risk scores that were not clinically validated. Most labs offering WGS or WES to physicians don't report the majority of known common disease variants.

Currently, the raw data from 23andMe are available to consumers, many of whom are taking that data and using software from Promethease (www .promethease.com) and other sites to generate health reports. Promethease is a literature retrieval system that builds a health report from genotypes based on scientific findings cited in SNPedia (www.snpedia.com), a wiki of curated human genetic associations from the scientific literature. These results are not as well vetted, curated, or communicated as 23andMe's, which invites a healthy degree of skepticism about the value of these reports.

RISKS AND BENEFITS TO SEQUENCING HEALTHY PEOPLE

There is no doubt that many patients are interested in knowing their genetic information, and for different reasons. It's important for health care providers to understand and respect this desire and the personal utility that one may realize from knowing their genome, even in the absence of established clinical utility. Research suggests that consumers who undertake personal genomic testing are interested in not just predicting future disease, but also motivated by finding out whether their existing conditions or traits have a genetic etiology[4].

There are several concerns with sequencing healthy individuals, some of which are augmented if those results are delivered by professionals without appropriate training[5].

Variants of uncertain significance (VUS)

First, even if a gene has been previously shown to be associated with a disease, many variants could be found in that gene that are novel. When found in symptomatic patients these variants are easier to interpret, but much less so in healthy persons, where the variant is likely to become a VUS.

Cost to follow-up positive findings

When a person tests positive for a known pathogenic variant and has no signs of disease, it may be tempting to look closer for signs of disease, even when the risk of disease is unclear. Most of the information we have about pathogenic variants has been obtained from studying people with the disease. The pathogenicity and penetrance (probability of disease) of these variants are often overestimated and need to be recalibrated using unselected cohorts before results are returned to patients. Under what circumstances should health care dollars be spent in pursuit of a disease for which the only risk factor is a genetic variant whose true penetrance is unknown[6]?

Misinterpretation and distress

Some have argued that the consumer will misinterpret results of genetic testing, leading to either false reassurance or the possibility of unnecessary medical procedures. According to research, comprehension of genetic test results varies by demographic characteristics, numeracy and genetic knowledge, and types and format of the genetic information presented[7]. This emphasizes the importance of *how* health care providers deliver risk information. Others argue that consumers will be subject to psychological distress and anxiety based on their genetic test results. However, empirical research has repeatedly shown no evidence of harm to consumers based on their genomic test results. In fact, many consumers make positive changes to their health behavior based on genetic findings, including changes to their diet and exercise (Table 11-1)[8].

Storing and reanalyzing genomic data

The final major challenge with WGS screening is keeping a patient's genome up to date and integrated with their health care. Current WGS yields static reports in a rapidly changing field. Even for the small number of patients who undergo WES/WGS for diagnostic purposes, storing and reanalyzing the data is not easy; imagine multiplying this across the healthy population! Ideally an individual's genomic sequence would be a living thing, constantly being reanalyzed in light of new knowledge, with poorly covered regions being filled as technology advances. This dynamic data would be incorporated into the individual's electronic health record

Table 11-1. Results from a survey on behavior change among people undergoing genomic testing in the PGEN Study.

Change	% of people reporting[a]
Dietary patterns	72
Exercise habits	61
Supplements (with medical consultation)	17
Supplements (without medical consultation)	21
Nonprescription drugs (with medical consultation)	10
Nonprescription drugs (without medical consultation)	7
Prescription drugs (with medical consultation)	11
Prescription drugs (without medical consultation)	2

[a] *Among the 42% of 1051 surveyed people reporting positive changes to their health behavior. (Data from Green RC, Farahany NA: Regulation: The FDA is overcautious on consumer genomics, Nature. 2014 Jan 16;505(7483):286-287)*

in a way where symptoms, medications, allergies, and nongenetic test and imaging results were constantly being cross-referenced to the genome and the physician alerted to actionable associations. Nothing like this is in current use.

KEY POINTS TO ADDRESS WITH OSTENSIBLY HEALTHY PATIENTS UNDERGOING GENOMIC SEQUENCING

- *Negative or indeterminate results:* There is a common misperception that all pathogenic variants for a disease can be identified with sequencing and that the clinical significance of every variant identified will be clear[9]. Negative or indeterminate results could mean that their disease is not genetic. It could also mean that the variants identified in their genome are not clearly associated with disease at present. Patients may tend to overinterpret these results as good news. Negative genetic findings do not mean that the patient is not at risk of disease. Genetic forms of complex diseases like breast cancer, for example, account for <10% of disease.

- *Positive results:* The average genome will yield 2–6 risk variants per person[2]. It's important to keep in mind that genetics reflects a person's potential, not their destiny. The collective knowledge of how specific genetic variants affect our health is still very limited at this stage. As more individuals are sequenced, it is becoming clear that in many cases, the risk of disease for what were once thought of as high penetrance gene variants is much less than what was previously thought.

- *Follow-up:* In some cases, it might make sense to do proactive iterative phenotyping—in other words, testing for signs of disease that weren't already obvious—in ostensibly healthy individuals with positive genetic testing results. For example, a healthy person finds they have a pathogenic variant for cardiac arrhythmia, a physician may choose to have the patient undergo an electrocardiogram (EKG). This decision must be made on a case-by-case basis, weighing the value of early detection against the cost (which will likely be borne by the patient) of following up a false positive result (or even a true positive that will never present clinically). These decisions should be made in the context of the overall profile of the patient, including their family history.

REFERENCES

1. Kaiser J. Who has your DNA—or wants it. *Science*. 2015;349:1475.
2. Dewey FE, Grove ME, Pan C, et al. Clinical interpretation and implications of whole-genome sequencing. *JAMA*. 2014;311:1035-1045.
3. Londin ER, Clark P, Sponziello M, Kricka LJ, Fortina P, Park JY. Performance of exome sequencing for pharmacogenomics. *Per Med*. 2014;12:109-115.
4. Meisel SF, Carere DA, Wardle J, et al. Explaining, not just predicting, drives interest in personal genomics. *Genome Med*. 2015;7:74.

5. Frueh FW, Greely HT, Green RC, Hogarth S, Siegel S. The future of direct-to-consumer clinical genetic tests. *Nat Rev Genet.* 2011;12:511-515.
6. Solomon BD. Incidentalomas in genomics and radiology. *N Engl J Med.* 2014;370:988-990.
7. Ostergren JE, Gornick MC, Carere DA, et al. How well do customers of direct-to-consumer personal genomic testing services comprehend genetic test results? Findings from the impact of personal genomics study. *Public Health Genomics.* 2015;18:216-224.
8. Green RC, Farahany NA. Regulation: the FDA is overcautious on consumer genomics. *Nature.* 2014;505:286-287.
9. Amendola LM, Lautenbach D, Scollon S, et al. Illustrative case studies in the return of exome and genome sequencing results. *Per Med.* 2015;12:283-295.

APPENDICES

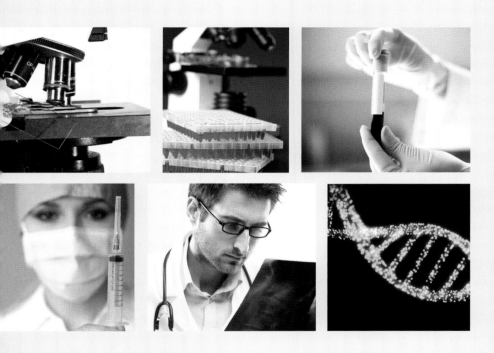

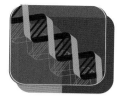

The Human Genome and Genetic Variation

The Human Genome Project has taught us a great deal about the different types of variations that exist in our genomes and their distribution across human populations. Humans are 99.9% identical at the DNA level, but the corollary is that at 0.1% of the nucleotide positions, translating to about 4–5 million basepairs on average, we differ[1]. These genetic differences will vary in their effect on human traits according to their location with respect to genes and their impact on the downstream proteins that those genes encode.

ORGANIZATION AND FUNCTION OF THE HUMAN GENOME

DNA

The human genome encompasses all of the DNA in an individual. This includes not only the nuclear DNA, but mitochondrial DNA as well. Mitochondrial DNA, as the name implies, is found in the mitochondria of each cell, is inherited only from the mother, and is usually considered separately from nuclear DNA. Nuclear DNA exists in the cell's nucleus, and is therefore found in every cell in the body that has a nucleus (pretty much all cells except red blood cells) and in each of these cells, the DNA is for the most part identical.

Chromosomes

The nuclear genome exists not as one long string of 3.2 billion nucleotides, but rather, it is broken into 23 discrete chunks, also known as chromosomes. Humans actually have two genomes, one from each parent, giving a total complement of 46 chromosomes, 22 pair of autosomes and one pair of sex chromosomes (X and Y). The size of DNA is measured in terms of the number of nucleotide *base pairs* (bp), or quantities of base pairs: kilobases (Kb = 1000 bp) and megabases (Mb = 10^6 bp).

The classic image of a karyotype (Fig. A1-1) depicts chromosomes as they appear during cell division, at which time the DNA condenses into a form called chromatin. Chromatin is the result of DNA wrapping around proteins, called histones. When in this form, chromosomes can be visualized under a light microscope. At other times, the DNA relaxes, unwinds from the histones, and reveals genes, regions of DNA that code for proteins. Genes in this state are accessible to cellular machinery that reads the DNA message and directs the production of proteins for the cell.

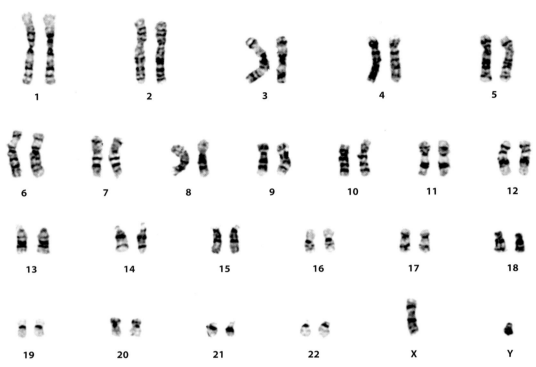

Figure A1-1. Karyotype depicting chromosomes as they appear during cell division. A normal karyotype has 22 pair of autosomes and one pair of sex chromosomes. This karyotype has sex chromosomes X and Y, indicating a male.

Genes and protein synthesis

While the DNA in every cell of the body is virtually identical, the proteins produced in those cells are not. Each cell is unique and differentiated, based on the complement of proteins it produces. Genes comprise only 1–2% of the human genome. The function of the remaining 98% of DNA is not fully understood at present, but includes many diverse functions, examples of which include ensuring structural stability of the chromosomes, regulating gene expression, and producing untranslated RNAs.

Protein synthesis involves transcription of the DNA code of the gene into messenger RNA (mRNA), followed by translation of the mRNA into protein (Fig. A1-2). The mRNA uses only certain parts of the gene, the exons, or coding region. The introns are portions of DNA that are removed. For many genes, the majority of the DNA between the beginning and the end of the gene is intron sequence!

The classic paradigm that one gene codes for one protein is not the norm. Instead, for 90% of genes, alternative forms of the protein can be made by splicing different exons of that gene together.

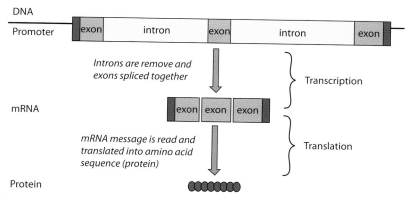

DNA

Promoter

mRNA

Protein

Introns are remove and exons spliced together

Transcription

mRNA message is read and translated into amino acid sequence (protein)

Translation

Figure A1-2. The process of protein synthesis. DNA is first transcribed into an intermediate molecule, messenger RNA (mRNA). In the process, segments of DNA are removed (introns) and the remaining pieces (exons) are spliced together to form the mature mRNA message. The mRNA is then translated into an amino acid sequence (protein).

Regulation of gene expression

If a cell were cracked open at any given time, one would find inside the entire human genome in DNA, but only the genes that are actually transcribed will be represented by mRNA. Thus, measuring mRNA transcripts can be a useful surrogate measure of which genes are turned on, or *expressed*, and making proteins. Regulation of gene expression is controlled via several mechanisms, including binding of specific regulatory molecules (either proteins, DNA or RNA) to regulatory regions of a gene. Other mechanisms include methylation, histone acetylation, and other forms of epigenetic modifications to the DNA. Epigenetics refers to chemical modifications to DNA that do not involve changes to the underlying sequence, but can still be inherited. These mechanisms effectively control which genes are making protein and which genes are not, at any given time for any given cell.

DNA VARIATION IN THE HUMAN GENOME

How do mutations arise?

Every cell in the body has virtually the same DNA sequence, which was inherited from each parent, carried by the sperm and egg. From the point of fertilization onward, the cells in the human body are continually dividing and during this process, the DNA must be replicated and transmitted to each daughter cell. The fidelity of this process is not perfect, leading to errors. Sometimes the wrong nucleotide, or an extra nucleotide, is added to the replicated DNA strand. Other times a nucleotide may be skipped, resulting in a small deletion. Other sources of errors include ionizing radiation, ultraviolet light, chemicals, and other mutagens, which induce DNA damage. In all cases, cellular repair mechanisms work to correct these errors, but occasionally they fail to do so and a mutation is born.

Random new mutations that arise in a single cell in the mature body are confined to that cell and the relatively few offspring of that cell when it subsequently divides. These *somatic* mutations typically have no measurable consequence on the function of the cell (the exception is in cancer, which is a disease of somatic mutations).

Mutations that are occur in the germ cells, the sperm or egg, will appear in every cell of that newly formed human being and are called *germline* mutations. The rate of new (de novo) germline mutations in humans is approximately 1×10^{-8} per bp per generation and therefore results in a newborn having on average 50–100 de novo mutations in their germline genome that aren't found in either parent. The vast majority of these will have no health consequences.

Different types of genetic variation, by size

There are many types of genetic variation, and they range in size from small, affecting single DNA nucleotides, to large, affecting entire chromosomes (Fig. A1-3). The largest type of variation is the aneuploidy, a numerical variant where entire chromosomes are either missing (monosomy) or an extra copy is present (trisomy). Few of these are viable and include the autosomal trisomies 13, 18, 21 and sex chromosome aneuploidies XXY, XO, XXX, and XYY. The next largest are the structural variants, defined as DNA variants ≥50 bp

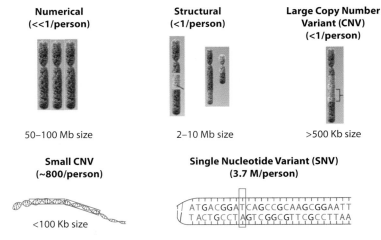

Figure A1-3. Different types of genetic variation, by size. Large genetic variants, like numerical (e.g., trisomies), structural (e.g., large deletions or translocations), or copy number variants are uncommon in an individual. The most prevalent type of genetic variation in a person involves single nucleotide positions.

in size and including insertions, deletions, duplications, and inversions of chromosomal regions. Copy number variant (CNV) are a type of structural variant involving hundreds of kilobases to megabases of DNA that are either missing or duplicated in tandem (sometimes multiple times). Most structural variants are individually rare, affecting <1/500 individuals, but there are about 1000 structural variants that are very common in the population, affecting one in two individuals[2]. The average person has about 2100–2500 structural variants in their genome. Larger structural variants are often very deleterious, involving many genes and are typically de novo (i.e., not inherited, but new mutations) and so large as to be visible under a microscope. Due to repetitive sequences in the genome that have a propensity to recombine, some deletions and duplication occur spontaneously more often than others. An example would be the deletion at 22q.11, which causes a variable syndrome with several names such as DiGeorge or velocardiofacial syndrome.

Variants involving fewer than 50 bp of DNA are more common in an individual and in the population. Single nucleotide variants (SNVs) and short insertions/deletions (InDels) make up the bulk of variants in a human genome, numbering at about 4–5 million per person[3].

CONSEQUENCES OF HUMAN GENOME VARIATION

The consequence of a given DNA variant depends in large part on whether it directly impacts a gene's ability to produce protein, that is, whether it results in the gene producing too much, too little, or a different protein than it's suppose to. Deviations from a normal level of gene expression, for example, decreased expression (termed haploinsufficiency) from a loss of a gene copy or increased expression (termed triplosensitivity) from gain of a gene copy is sufficient to cause disease in some cases. For other genes, missing or extra copies has no overt effect on health. Numerical, structural, and large CNVs have the greatest potential to do damage because they affect the largest number of genes. Extra copies of genes can result in overexpression of the gene products, while too few copies can result in underexpression. Translocations and inversions can result in fusion genes, hybrids formed from two genes that come into proximity following the structural rearrangement. These fusion genes can result in a product whose function is new or different from the two fusion partners.

Small CNVs and SNVs have variable effects ranging from completely innocuous to highly deleterious, depending on where they occur. Since genes comprise <2% of the genome, most of these variants will occur in nongenic regions and will likely be innocuous. Small CNVs that result in deletion or duplication of entire genes or portions of genes are more likely to be deleterious compared to those that do not involve genes. Even those variants that occur in genes may not have an effect unless they are in a coding, splice site, or regulatory region.

SNVs are the most well-studied type of variation. The most prevalent type of SNV is a single nucleotide substitution (e.g., a C replaces a T in a given

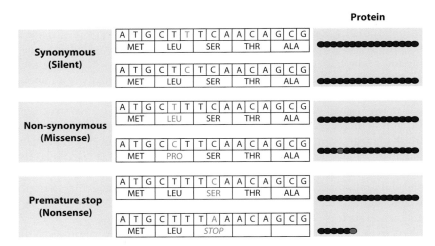

Figure A1-4. Consequences to proteins as the result of single nucleotide changes in DNA. The effect of single nucleotide variants on protein structure can range from no effect on the amino acid composition (synonymous), to a change of one amino acid (nonsynonymous), to a change in the length of the protein due to a premature stop signal being introduced.

position). These substitutions are considered *silent* if they do not change the amino acid of the resulting protein (aka *synonymous*) (Fig. A1-4). If they do change the amino acid, they are called *missense* variants (aka *nonsynonymous*). They can also change the amino acid to a stop codon (aka *nonsense*), leading to premature truncation of the protein (*stop gained*) or in some cases the loss of a stop signal (*stop loss*). Less prevalent are small InDels, which typically have the effect of shifting the reading frame and disrupting the entire protein sequence downstream of the variant, including premature stops or protein length changes. SNVs occurring in splice sites can interfere with joining of the exons during transcription, resulting in different protein transcripts. Protein length changing variants (frameshift, stop loss or gain) or those that affect splicing are considered the most damaging, often leading to a loss of function of the gene. The average genome has about 149–182 of these[3].

PATTERNS OF GENETIC VARIATION ACROSS POPULATIONS

A specific genetic variant typically arises in a single individual, the founder, who then passes the variant down to subsequent generations. The frequency of the variant in the population (also called the allele frequency) is a measure of how many people have the variant and is shaped by several factors, including any effect on reproductive fitness (the extreme being lethality), and even chance. In general, the more deleterious the variant is, the lower the allele frequency will be in the population. Variants are sometimes classified based on their allele frequency, as either rare, low frequency, or common. A common

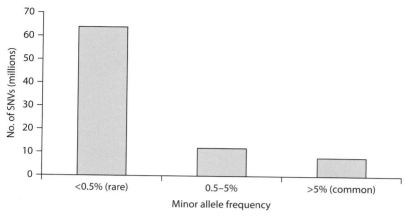

Figure A1-5. Relative abundance of single nucleotide variants by their allele frequency. A rare variant is one that is found in very few individuals (<5/1000) in the population. Common variants are found in >5% of people. It is thought that nearly all of the approximately 8 million common variants have been discovered, while the number of rare variants (currently at about 65 million) continues to grow as more individuals are sequenced.

variant is one that, if you sampled 1000 people in the population, you would find at least 50 people carrying that variant. In contrast, a rare variant would be found in <5/1000 individuals in the population. Collectively, rare variants are the most abundant type, with over 60 million of them described to date (Fig. A1-5). That they are rare may be an indication that they are young, introduced into the population only relatively recently. Population dynamics like the breeding and migration patterns of the local population to which the person acquiring the mutation belongs also impacts the allele frequency. Indeed, the historical migration of people has shaped the global distribution of variants, resulting in distinct differences in allele frequencies by continent, race, and ethnicity.

While the allele frequencies of many genomic variants do vary by race and ethnicity, the idea that the major racial groups have a distinct genetic signature that defines them is incorrect. Overall genetic differences between individuals within a racial group can be greater than the differences between the races. In general genetic variation is distributed in a continuous, overlapping fashion between geographically distinct populations, consistent with migration patterns of early humans.

RESOURCES

DbSNP (www.ncbi.nlm.nih.gov/SNP/)

Catalogue of variation in humans and other species, hosted by the NCBI and NHGRI

1000 Genomes Project (www.1000genomes.org/)

This allele frequency database from the NIH is derived from whole genome and targeted exome sequencing of about 2500 individuals from 26 populations.

Exome Variant Server (EVS) (evs.gs.washington.edu/EVS/)

This allele frequency database comes from the exome sequencing project (ESP) of the National Heart Lung and Blood Institute (NHLBI). Allele frequencies were derived from exome sequencing of about 6500 individuals who were part of various large well-phenotyped cohorts in the United States.

Exome Aggregation Consortium (ExAc) (exac.broadinstitute.org/)

This allele frequency database from the Broad Institute is derived from sequencing of >60,706 individuals from various disease-specific and population genetic studies.

REFERENCES

1. 1000 Genomes Project Consortium, Auton A, Brooks LD, et al. A global reference for human genetic variation. *Nature.* 2015;526:68-74.
2. Sudmant PH, Rausch T, Gardner EJ, et al. An integrated map of structural variation in 2,504 human genomes. *Nature.* 2015;526:75-81.
3. UK10K Consortium, Walter K, Min JL, et al. The UK10K project identifies rare variants in health and disease. *Nature.* 2015;526:82-90.

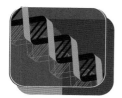

Laboratory Methods to Detect Genome Variation

There are a variety of clinical laboratory testing methods in use, each with its different applications, strengths, and limitations. Different types of genomic variation require different methodologies to detect them. Specific clinical applications may sometimes require the use of multiple methodologies to be comprehensive, sometimes used in parallel, other times sequentially. With technological advances, current methodologies may be supplanted with newer ones because they are faster, cheaper, and/or higher throughput. In general, the following guide will be useful for matching the methodology to the type of variation it can detect, and providing practical advice for the use of genomic testing modalities. First, we would like to clarify some terms commonly used for testing.

TARGETED (GENOTYPING) VERSUS NONTARGETED METHODS

Targeted methods typically referred to as genotyping, analyze only specific, known DNA variants while nontargeted methods are more comprehensive and allow for the discovery of new DNA variants. In other words, one must already know what genetic variant one is looking for in the case of a targeted genotyping test, usually because the variant is a known cause of the disease. An example would be the factor V Leiden variant that confers an increased risk of thrombosis. Advantages of targeted genotyping are the lower cost and more rapid turnaround time. A disadvantage is that targeted tests may miss detecting genetic changes that are not suspected a priori.

Laboratory tests range from measuring a single analyte to a group of analytes to the entire complement of analytes (for DNA, this is the whole genome). Terminology that captures multiplex or genome-wide analysis includes panels, array, and microarray.

The following are descriptions of commonly used technologies in genomic medicine.

CHROMOSOME STUDIES

Karyotyping

Karyotyping is a nontargeted cytogenetic technique used to detect chromosomal numerical variants (aneuploidies), large copy number variants (deletions or insertions), and structural variants across the genome (translocations, inversions). As such, a karyotype can be a screening test, looking for any change in the chromosomes that might cause a disease, or a diagnostic test, analyzing for a particular trisomy, for example.

A variety of tissues can be analyzed by karyotyping, including blood (i.e., lymphocytes), fibroblasts (usually from a skin biopsy), amniocytes (from amniocentesis), chorionic villi, products of conception, and tumor cells. Cells are captured during mitosis when the chromosomes are condensed, and the chromosomes are chemically fixed, stained, and then spread out on a slide. The most commonly used stain is Giemsa, also called GTG or G-banding. This staining labels some regions of the chromosomes darker (usually rich in A and T bases, generally indicating less gene-rich areas) and lighter areas (richer in G and C, usually with more genes). Images of the chromosomes from single cells are taken and analyzed with software that allows all the chromosome pairs to be viewed individually and aligned with each other. In the most critical step, a trained cytogeneticist must manually examine the chromosome images to determine if the number of chromosomes is correct, if the banding patterns are normal, and if any abnormalities are detected, what chromosome regions are involved. This can be tricky. For example, a translocation involving a single band might be visible, but it may be challenging to determine what chromosome the extra band came from, which could be very important to predict the possible health implications of the chromosomal abnormality. Newer technologies like arrays (see below) can address these challenges.

Depending on the phase of mitosis and the condensation of the chromosomes when they are fixed, karyotypes can yield between approximately 400 and 800 bands, which limits the ability to visualize changes in chromosomal segments to those >5 Mb in size, though this exact number varies across chromosomes based on the complexity of the banding patterns.

Chromosomal nomenclature

The terminology used to describe changes in chromosomes is described by the International System for Human Cytogenetic Nomenclature. Terminologies range from simple (normal is 46,XX or 46,XY) to highly complex and esoteric. A few generalities are helpful to know:

- The first number is the total number of chromosomes. For germline samples this number will be close to 46 (normal), while it can be highly variable for cancer samples.

- The next characters are the sex chromosomes, which can be XX (normal female), XY (normal male), XXY (Klinefelter), XYY, XXX, or several other combinations of additional sex chromosomes. Turner syndrome is denoted 45,X. *Not 45,XO.*

- Extra chromosomes are simply indicated with a + sign, as in 47,XX +21.

- If a region of a chromosome is referred to, the nomenclature starts with the chromosome number (1–22), the arm of the chromosome (p for the short arm, q for the long arm), and then the band and sub-band.

For example, 1p36 refers to the short arm of chromosome one, band 3, sub-band 6. Note that 6 is a sub-band of 3, so the correct way to read this is "one p three six" not "one p thirty-six."

Common and appropriate uses of karyotyping include the evaluation of known or suspected trisomies before or after birth, such as after a positive prenatal screen or in a baby with features consistent with Trisomy 21, or to detect physical translocations or other large structural alterations. As a screening test for most phenotypes (e.g., developmental delay), karyotyping has been largely supplanted by array technologies. It is highly uncommon for there to be pathogenic chromosomal alterations that are detectable by karyotype but not array. Nevertheless, the structural information provided by a karyotype cannot be fully replicated by any other technology, and karyotyping remains an important tool. Limitations of arrays that are complemented by karyotyping are discussed below.

> **Key Point**
>
> As a first-pass screening test for nonspecific conditions (e.g., dysmorphic features or developmental delay), karyotypes have been largely replaced by array technologies, though the karyotype remains an important test.

Fluorescence in situ hybridization (FISH)

FISH is also a cytogenetic technique, but is used for targeted identification of specific predefined chromosomal abnormalities (see targeted methods above). FISH uses fluorescent probes designed to bind to specific chromosomal regions and then visualized under a fluorescence microscope. It can detect lesions as small as 50–100 kb in size. It is used in the diagnosis of subchromosomal abnormalities causing diseases like Prader–Willi/Angelman syndrome (deletion on 15q), Cri-du-chat syndrome (deletion involving 5p), and 22q11 deletion syndrome (DiGeorge). Probes targeting sequence on a particular chromosome can also be used to count that chromosome and thus identify aneuploides, particularly those that are viable (13, 18, 21, X, Y), and can be done more rapidly and can better detect mosaicism by analyzing more cells than karyotyping. Additionally, probes at the ends of chromosomes (subtelomeric) can be used to identify translocations or copy number changes involving the ends of chromosomes. The key concept for FISH is that it is not a comprehensive screening test and only tests for the presence, absence, and copy number of the region selected.

FISH Nomenclature:

- nuc ish indicates the FISH was performed on an intact nucleus, while ish indicates that the chromosomes were spread out.

- For aneuploidies, the probes are listed with the copy number (×2 is normal for autosomes) listed next to them.

Comparative genomic hybridization and SNP arrays

Arrays are a nontargeted method used to identify copy number variants in the whole genome. Two technologies are currently in use: comparative genomic

Important if considering a mosaic disorder. Was the right tissue tested?

It is highly recommended to provide clinical information if possible.

ISCN = International System for Human Cytogenetic Nomenclature. This designation is the "official" result of the array, providing the coordinates of the copy change and the nature of the copy change. x2 is normal for autosomes. x3 is a copy gain, x1 is a copy loss.

This is the expert's review, and the detail and effort will vary the most among different labs. The discussion will attempt to connect any detected variants with the reported phenotype (if provided).

Summary of findings. Significance can be benign, likely benign, uncertain, likely pathogenic, and pathogenic. The coordinates are specific to one genome build (see below).

This guidance is usually very general. Obtaining parental arrays to clarify an uncertain variant is usually a good practice.

Very important! The coordinates noted under the ISCN designation above are specific to the genome build.

The nitty-gritty, which is important. Gives size cutoffs for resolution and reporting. Smaller variants might be reported if the lab knows to pay attention to a particular genomic region or gene. When possible, provide clinical details and genes of interest.

A good review of the technical limitations of array technology. Arrays don't detect everything and reviewing any clinical suspicions with a specialist or the lab can help determine if they might be missed by an array.

Sample Type: Peripheral blood - EDTA
Clinical History: _____
SNP array
ISCN: arr 9q22.31(95,460,764–95,700,701)x3

If this array had been normal it would have also read "(XY)x1 indicating normal for male chromosomes. Sex chromosomes are not called if there is an abnormality on an array.

LABORATORY PHYSICIAN INTERPRETATION:
Male with variant of uncertain significance (copy gain within 9q22.31)
Unclear male result with interstitial duplication within 9q22.31 of uncertain clinical significance. Within this small ~0.33 Mb 9q22.31 region, there are 2 OMIM genes (CENPP, BICD2), 2 other protein-coding genes without well-characterized function (ZNF484, IPPK), and 5 pseudogenes (see below). Of these genes, only BICD2 (OMIM: 609797) has a characterized disease association, where heterozygous missense mutations are associated with autosomal dominant lower extremity-predominant spinal muscular atrophy-2 (SMALED2; OMIM: 615290). No similar duplications have been described in any of the searched databases (ClinGen and DECIPHER describing the affected population, DGV describing the normal population). Therefore, it is uncertain whether this duplication is a benign variant or carries any clinical significance based on currently available data.

Unclear Finding:
1) 9q22.31 Copy Gain
Genomic Coordinates: 95,460,764-95,700,701
Estimated Size: 0.340 Mb
Number of Probes: 57 Probes
Significance: Uncertain clinical significance
Inheritance: Unknown
Genes: CENPP, IPPK, BICD2, ANKRD19P, RNU6-714P, EEF1DP2, ZNF484, SNX18P2, ALOX15P2

Unclear results are a common outcome of high-resolution tests like arrays, which must be considered and counseled before an array is sent, including the possible need for parental testing.

Size plays an important role in suggesting pathogenicity. Deletions/duplications >1 Mb are concerning and >3 Mb are likely to be pathogenic. These are generalizations.

GUIDANCE FOR NEXT STEPS:
1) Parental analyses could be considered to clarify whether these copy number changes were de novo or inherited from a carrier parent.
2) Genetic counseling is recommended.
3) Clinical correlation is required.

RESOURCES FOR PHYSICIANS:
1) UCSC genome browser at http://genome.ucsc.edu/cgi-bin/hgGateway
2) Online Mendelian Inheritance in Man at http://www.ncbi.nlm.nih.gov/omim
3) DECIPHER: Database of Chromosomal Imbalance and Phenotype in Humans using Ensembl Resources. Firth, HV, et al. *Am J Hum Genet.* 2009;84:524–533. doi: dx.doi.org/10/1016/j.ajhg.2009.03.010 at http://decipher.sanger.ac.uk
4) Database of Genomic Variants at http://dgv.tcag.ca/dgv/app/home
5) Clinical Genome Resource (ClinGen) www.clinicalgenome.org

REFERENCES:

The lab may provide references for their clinical conclusions that may be directly relevant to patient counseling and management. There may be more important references not cited by the lab!

The technology used to perform the array and the number of probes. More probes = higher resolution and more small uncertain variants.

METHODOLOGY:
Whole genome single nucleotide polymorphism-based cytogenomic array (SNP array) was performed using the Illumina CytoSNP-850K Platform with genome build hg19 to detect genome-wide genomic copy number changes (CNVs) and regions of homozygosity (ROH). This array platform contains over 850,000 SNPs in 15x redundancy throughout the genome with enriched coverage for 3262 genes of known relevance in both constitutional and cancer applications. The average probe spacing across the whole array is approximately 1.8 kb. CNVs in the backbone of the genome involving less than 16 contiguous probes are not reported. Therefore, the overall effective resolution across the whole array is approximately 29.0 kb. Involvement of a minimum of 12 contiguous probes is required to report a CNV in a critical gene/locus. Benign and likely benign CNVs as well as CNVs less than 1 Mb with unknown clinical significance but without involvement of annotated disease-causing genes are not reported for the prenatal testing. For postnatal testing, CNVs <200 kb are not reported unless there is strong evidence of pathogenicity. Classification of clinical significance of CNVs is based on the ACMGG standards and guidelines [Kearney et al. American College of Medical Genetics standards and guidelines for interpretation and reporting of postnatal constitutional copy number variants. *Genet Med.* 2011; 13(7):680–685].

DISCLAIMER:
SNP array is designed to identify CNVs associated with genomic imbalances, as well as ROH. This test will detect aneuploidy, triploidy, deletions, duplications, and ROH of the loci represented on the microarray utilized. It will not detect balanced genomic rearrangements, imbalances and ROH of regions not represented on the microarray. It may not detect tetraploidy caused by endoduplication. The detection level for an alteration may vary depending on the locus. Failure to detect an alteration (gain or loss) at any disease-causing locus/gene does not exclude the diagnosis of any of the disorders associated with the locus/gene, since other mutation mechanisms may lead to the diagnosis. Some unrecognized potential pathogenic CNVs may be classified as unknown clinical significance or nonpathogenic at the time of analysis based on available data. This assay may detect mosaicism of >30% in nonmixed specimens with optimal DNA quality. Mosaicism may not be detected in specimens with mixed cells/tissues (such as prenatal specimens mixed with maternal cells) and specimens with suboptimal DNA quality. This assay may detect maternal cell contamination (MCC) or chimerism in prenatal specimens, which may result in noninformative results for copy number variants and ROH. Copy number variants and ROH below the cut-off thresholds established in this lab are not reported, unless evidence supports the variant or ROH is pathologic. The lab will report ROH detected in known imprinted regions/chromosomes, which may indicate pathogenic uniparental disomy (UPD). UPD suggested by ROH must be verified by a different method. In addition, ROH may indicate increased risk of expression of recessive mutations. However, it may also reveal consanguinity or inbreeding. The lab will not report ROH that is not related to the known imprinted regions/chromosomes unless a written request with a consent form for releasing such findings is signed by the patient, and the lab is not liable for any legal issues related to releasing such findings.

hybridization (CGH) and single nucleotide polymorphism (SNP) arrays; the latter is rapidly supplanting the former, though SNP arrays themselves will likely be replaced by next-generation sequencing (NGS) technologies in the coming years.

Array CGH is performed by shredding a patient's entire genome, labeling these small DNA fragments with a fluorescent color, and then annealing the small DNA fragments to a chip that contains hundreds of thousands of oligonucleotides corresponding to approximately regularly spaced regions in the genome. A reference sample of similarly shredded, differently colored DNA is applied at the same time, and the two genomes literally compete to bind the oligonucleotides on the chip's surface. Regions in the patient's genome that are deleted will not compete as well, and regions that are duplicated will compete better for oligonucleotides than the reference sample. By comparing the relative hybridization of the two genomes, one can identify copy number variations relative to the reference.

SNP arrays also start by shredding the patient's DNA, but no fluorescent labeling or comparison DNA is needed. Instead, the oligonucleotides on the chip surface are designed to end one base before known common SNPs in the human genome. Fluorescent DNA bases are added and only the base corresponding to the base in the patient's DNA is added at each position. Extra and missing DNA can now be detected in two ways. First, fewer bases are added in regions of the genome with a missing copy, and this absolute change can be detected (unlike the relative change in a CGH array). Second, because most people have mixed ancestries and therefore are heterozygous for many common SNPs, whenever a region loses heterozygosity this suggests a deletion because only one version of each SNP is detected. Overall, SNP arrays are slightly higher resolution and are more robust at identifying deletions and duplications than CGH arrays. There is no reason to use a CGH array if a SNP array is available. On the other hand, if a patient was tested with a CGH array that was normal, the yield from repeating the test with an SNP array is probably very low.

Other advantages of SNP arrays over CGH include the ability of SNP arrays to detect some forms of uniparental disomy, which can be a cause of diseases associated with abnormal imprinting (such as Prader–Willi, though SNP array is not 100% sensitive for this disorder). SNP arrays can also be useful for detecting areas of homozygosity caused by consanguinity. This information can be helpful when trying to shorten a list of potential genetic causes of recessive disorders, but can be unwanted information and it is appropriate to counsel patients that this test will identify if the patient's parents are related. Rarely, SNP arrays have been reported to identify cases of incest that led to challenging legal-ethical situations.

The resolution of arrays depends in part on the spacing between the probes (which can be as little as 10 kb), and the guidelines of the laboratory for reporting variants (usually only >200 kb, or a certain number of probes in known genes). The reason for not reporting smaller variants, particularly those in regions not known to cause disease, is that the number of false positive (i.e., noise rather than true deletions or duplications) or variant of uncertain significance (VUS) results increase dramatically as smaller and smaller variants are reported. Improvements and standardization of these reporting criteria are likely to change rapidly.

> **Key Point**
>
> Do not ignore VUSs, even though they are frustrating. Ideally each should be researched further in the literature or in the family. At the very least they should remain a part of the patient's medical record until more information becomes available to better classify each uncertain variant. Evaluation of a VUS remains an important role for genetics professionals.

Like with karyotyping, the most critical step in the application of array technologies is the review by a trained specialist of the findings on the array. This specialist will not only rely on software to identify copy number variants, but also will manually review the entire genome for areas that might have changes in copy number, particularly those involving genes that might be relevant to the patient's phenotype (assuming this information is provided). The specialist will then review a number of databases including DGV (http://dgv.tcag.ca/), DECIPHER (https://decipher.sanger.ac.uk/), and ClinGen (http://www.ncbi.nlm.nih.gov/projects/dbvar/clingen/), and major genome browsers (genome.ucsc.edu/) to determine if a detected CNV has been previously observed, and if so, was it observed in normal individuals or in patients with phenotypes consistent with that of the person being tested. The specialist will also review the genes in each CNV to determine if any evidence exists that changes in these genes might cause disease. Variants with some associated data are interpreted as being benign, likely benign, likely pathogenic, or pathogenic. Very importantly, it is often the case that insufficient evidence exists to link a CNV to the patient's phenotype, and this CNV will be categorized as a VUS.

> **Key Point**
>
> Array reports from diagnostic laboratories should not be viewed as representing exhaustive research of detected variants. There are limited standards for the depth and type of research into detected variants. The ordering practitioner must often delve further to make management decisions.

The depth of database research that goes into assigning pathogenicity to a variant and the final judgment of the individual reviewing the array are both *subjective and variable* across experts and labs. The expert review of an array is not the final word and may not be sufficient to translate the results of the array into concrete medical decisions. Any practitioner ordering genomic testing must take responsibility for evaluating the results, critically assessing the literature used to support the report's diagnosis (or lack thereof), and considering if further evaluation of uncertain findings is needed.

Array technologies do have some important limitations. Because the genome is shredded in order to perform any array test, all position information is lost. Additional detected DNA (copy gains) can be anywhere in the genome. Depending on the size of the duplicated region, karyotyping, FISH, or sequencing may be required to clarify the location of the additional DNA if such information would be clinically useful, though this is generally not the case. For example, any patient with a deletion or duplication detected on array that involves the end of a chromosome should undergo a karyotype to determine if that change involves a translocation, and in most cases the parents should undergo karyotyping as well.

In time, the same concept that uses SNP genotyping to infer copy number will likely be extended to NGS and arrays will fall out of use. Instead, selected regions of the genome will be sequenced in sufficient depth to determine zygosity and copy number. This way, the same technology will be used for identifying sequence variants or copy number variants.

> **Key Point**
>
> Rather than a first-line screen, karyotypes are often used to clarify the results of an array, such as to determine if terminal deletions or duplications involve a translocation, which is critical for determining recurrence risk.

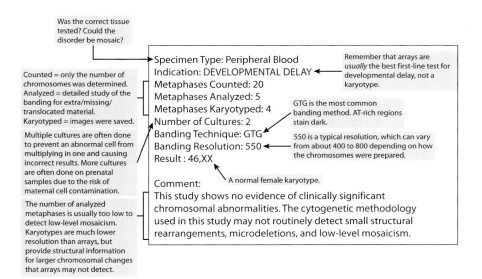

Was the correct tissue tested? Could the disorder be mosaic?

Counted = only the number of chromosomes was determined. Analyzed = detailed study of the banding for extra/missing/translocated material. Karyotyped = images were saved.

Multiple cultures are often done to prevent an abnormal cell from multiplying in one and causing incorrect results. More cultures are often done on prenatal samples due to the risk of maternal cell contamination.

The number of analyzed metaphases is usually too low to detect low-level mosaicism. Karyotypes are much lower resolution than arrays, but provide structural information for larger chromosomal changes that arrays may not detect.

Specimen Type: Peripheral Blood
Indication: DEVELOPMENTAL DELAY
Metaphases Counted: 20
Metaphases Analyzed: 5
Metaphases Karyotyped: 4
Number of Cultures: 2
Banding Technique: GTG
Banding Resolution: 550
Result : 46,XX

Comment:
This study shows no evidence of clinically significant chromosomal abnormalities. The cytogenetic methodology used in this study may not routinely detect small structural rearrangements, microdeletions, and low-level mosaicism.

Remember that arrays are *usually* the best first-line test for developmental delay, not a karyotype.

GTG is the most common banding method. AT-rich regions stain dark.

550 is a typical resolution, which can vary from about 400 to 800 depending on how the chromosomes were prepared.

A normal female karyotype.

SEQUENCING TESTS AND TECHNOLOGIES

Targeted genotyping of single nucleotide variants

There are various methods in use, such as the Taqman® method, which takes advantage of the 5'-nuclease assay chemistry of Taq polymerase and uses fluorescently labeled allele-specific probes to distinguish different genotypes. Taqman® is widely used for custom analysis of individual variants. Targeted genotyping can also be performed across large numbers of variants simultaneously using multiplex genotyping arrays. These arrays are designed to analyze from several hundred to a million or more preselected SNVs across the genome. Arrays are used more often for research, for example, in genome-wide association studies. They are also an efficient way to provide health information across a wide range of conditions (e.g., the 23andMe test) or highly polymorphic gene panels (e.g., drug metabolizing enzymes or human leukocyte antigens).

Sanger sequencing (aka dideoxy-sequencing)

This older sequencing technology is still widely used, and useful, in the clinical setting. In brief, a patient's DNA is targeted with a primer at the site of interest, and new DNA bases are added at the end of the primer. A small percentage of the bases are chemically modified so that they are fluorescent (one color for each of the four bases) and terminate the DNA chain once added. After many rounds elongating the original primer, the result is many different length DNA molecules that are synthesized complementary to the patient's DNA, each ending with a fluorescent base indicating the base at that position. By resolving the strands, the sequence can be directly read.

Sanger sequencing has several major advantages. It produces high-quality sequence that can extend up to about 800 bases, compared to next-generation technologies that mostly produce read lengths of <200 bases with higher error rates (hence the need for deeper coverage, see below). It is also cheap when used at smaller scales and can be easily targeted to nearly any position in the genome without having to manipulate the patient's DNA. Sanger sequencing is therefore the method of choice for sequencing small numbers of genes with high quality, or analyzing single locations in the genome. Most single-gene tests and small panels are conducted with Sanger sequencing, and many labs use Sanger sequencing to improve the coverage of larger gene panels due to regions that are not sequenced well by next-generation approaches. Sanger sequencing, because it produces longer reads, is also useful for mapping breakpoints in chromosomal translocations or deletions, or determining if nearby mutations are on the same or different chromosomes (phase).

As the number of targets to be sequenced increases, Sanger sequencing becomes less efficient and less cost-effective because a new reaction is required for every about 800 bases. Sanger sequencing can detect mosaicism down to about 15%, while next-generation approaches, with sufficient depth, can be much more sensitive.

Next-generation sequencing (whole genome, whole exome, enrichment panels)

Next-generation sequencing refers to a group of technologies that produce thousands to millions of sequences simultaneously. Current clinical applications of NGS include analysis of human genetic variation for diagnostic or pre-disposition testing. These applications really employ *resequencing*, as opposed to de novo sequencing, since the reference human genome has already been assembled. In this case, a patient's DNA sequence is compared to the reference genome to determine what variation exists in that patient. Without relying on this reference sequencing, the process of assembling the patient's DNA would be far more laborious and likely prohibitive. The following steps are involved in resequencing for the purpose of identifying single nucleotide substitutions and small in/dels.

Enrichment

For some applications (whole exome and gene panels), a DNA sample is first subjected to an enrichment step that selects only a portion of the genome to analyze. In the case of whole-exome sequencing (WES), the exons (coding region) of the genome are captured. In the case of panels, a subset of genes is captured. It should be noted that exome capture is not foolproof and fails to capture all gene regions of the genome. In the case of panels, coverage of the specific genes is usually very good (e.g., hereditary cancer panel, neonatal epilepsy panel), either because the smaller number of genes permits better optimization of the capture method, or because Sanger sequencing is used to complete any gaps.

Sequence generation

The most commonly used sequencing technology today is from Illumina, inc. Their technology generates sequence information from genomic DNA that has been sheared into fragments that range in size from tens to hundreds of base pairs. Sequence generation occurs in a massively parallel fashion, from millions of DNA fragment templates from a single test sample all at once. Essentially what occurs is millions of DNA molecules from the patient are immobilized on a surface, a single fluorescent base is added to all DNA fragments, a high-resolution picture is taken of all these molecules, and the cycle repeats. The end result is a stack of about 50–250 images comprised of millions of colored dots, and the sequential colors of each dot represents its sequence. After the test sample fragments are sequenced, they are aligned to the human reference genome.

Alignment to reference genome

There is no "normal" or "control" human genome, there are billions of different genomes. To provide some sort of standard, a reference genome has been assembled, representing a mosaic of DNA from over a dozen anonymous volunteers. There are continual improvements in the reference sequence, but there are some gaps in difficult to sequence regions. Moreover, the reference genome may contain important variants of health significance that are not necessarily normal. For example, the current reference genome contains the factor V Leiden variant, associated with thrombophilia.

Importantly, the reference genome is constantly being updated, with major changes every few years. When reviewing results of a genomic test, it is essential to ensure that the version of the genome used to generate the test report (will always be indicated on the report) is the same as that being used to review the results on a genome browser or in the literature. Most tests done today use hg19 (aka GRCh37), which was released in 2009, or hg38 (GRCh38) released in 2013. Similarly, when communicating the location of a variant to a colleague or expert, it is important to include the reference genome version.

Variant calling

Anywhere that the test sequence differs from the reference genome will be considered a variant and appear as such in the standard variant call format (VCF) file. The quality of each variant is determined in large part by the *coverage*, in other words, how many DNA fragments were sequenced that overlap the variant location. The higher the coverage, the more confident the variant call. In general, genome-wide average coverage of 30× and site-specific coverage of at least 15–20× is desirable[1]. Each laboratory generally determines their own quality metrics, and these are major sources of variation among clinical labs performing NGS. It is expected that the U.S. Food and Drug Administration (FDA), the Clinical Laboratory Improvement Act of 1988 (CLIA), and professional organizations will work toward standardizing these variables in the coming years.

Once a variant file is produced, it can be analyzed using a number of bioinformatic tools. Standard genome interpretation involves first annotating the genome with information about the variant's location, especially relative to genes. The consequence of gene variants on the downstream protein is predicted and the frequency of the variant is determined from public variant databases. Further analyses depend on the specific application.

NGS for copy number variants

CNVs can be detected from whole-genome sequencing by evaluating the density of aligned reads along the genome. Originally this was difficult to perform, but bioinformatics approaches have improved. At this moment, however, NGS is not necessarily the gold standard to detect small copy number variants, which must be kept in mind when interpreting test results. The performance of NGS against other methodologies (e.g., array) to detect copy number variants should become more clear in the coming years but is expected to make major strides.

Long-read sequencing technology

Next-generation devices that produce long reads (10+ kb compared to 200 bases) are not yet used clinically but are an area of active research. Platforms include those developed by Pacific Biosciences (Menlo Park,

CA), Oxford Nanopore Technologies (Oxford, UK) and others. Long read technologies offer several advantages over traditional short read NGS. First, they provide structural information and can detect copy number variants and translocations with much better sensitivity. They can also detect phase, which refers to the presence of two changes on the same chromosome (cis) or one on each chromosome (trans). Determination of phase is particularly critical to diseases presumed to be recessive and is one of several reasons why including parental DNA in exome analysis improves yield.

ADDITIONAL TESTING METHODS

Quantitative real-time polymerase chain reaction (QRTPCR)—For analysis of RNA

QRTPCR (also abbreviated qPCR) is a targeted, quantitative method to measure the amount of RNA in a tissue to assess the level of gene expression. As a first step, the RNA in a tissue is converted to complementary DNA (cDNA), which is then used in the analysis. The analysis is based upon the polymerase chain reaction (PCR), a technique used to amplify, or make copies of, DNA. Conventionally, PCR is a qualitative process, but in QRTPCR, the amplification process is monitored in real time and calibrated against a reference, often expression of other well-characterized genes, to determine a relative level of gene expression. Newer digital methods can provide an absolute quantification of the target DNA. This method can be used to analyze a single gene (e.g., ALK gene expression in cancer) or as a multiplex assay to measure the expression of several genes simultaneously (e.g., Oncotype Dx®).

Immunohistochemistry (IHC)—For analysis of proteins

IHC is a targeted method to measure the presence or absence of specific proteins in a tissue or cell. It is commonly utilized to localize these proteins in formalin-fixed, paraffin-embedded (FFPE) tissues. The technique exploits the binding of antibodies to specific protein sequences (antigens). Fluorescent tags or enzymatic reactions are used to be able to visualize the antibody bound to the protein under a light microscope. While the procedure is qualitative in nature, it becomes quantitative when used to assess what proportion of cells in a given tissue have the protein (e.g., the percent of cells that test positive). Common examples of the use of IHC include measuring estrogen and progesterone receptors in gynecological tumors.

Table A2-1 summarizes different clinical testing methods that a practitioner may come across, with the types of variant that can be detected and the ideal test for each.

Table A2-1. Clinical testing methods used for detecting variation in DNA, RNA, and protein.

Variation	Test(s) with some yield or low-throughput	Preferred test(s)
DNA variation		
Numerical/large structural changes of chromosomes	FISH (must know target), next-gen sequencing, SNP array	Karyotype
Deletions or duplications (megabases in size)	Karyotyping, FISH (must know target)	SNP array
Small CNVs (about kilobase size or smaller)	SNP array (depends on probe density)	Whole-genome sequencing
	Sanger sequencing (must know target)	Multiplex ligation-dependent probe amplification (MPLA)
	Whole-exome sequencing	Targeted array
SNVs (substitutions, in/dels)	Sanger sequencing (excellent if known target)	Targeted genotyping assays such as TaqMan (many others)
		Genotyping arrays
		Whole-genome sequencing
		Whole-exome sequencing (for exonic SNVs)
Other variation		
RNA expression	Quantitative PCR	Expression microarrays (research)
		Next-gen RNA sequencing (research)
Protein variation	IHC	Proteomics (research)
Epigenetic variation		Bisulfite sequencing (research)
		Methylation-specific restriction digestion (available clinically only for certain genes and applications)

REFERENCE

1. Meynert AM, Ansari M, FitzPatrick DR, Taylor MS. Variant detection sensitivity and biases in whole genome and exome sequencing. *BMC Bioinformatics*. 2014;15:247.

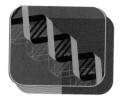

The Genetic Basis of Disease

The average human has approximately 4 million germline variants, that is, positions in their genome that differ from the reference genome (see Appendix 2 for a discussion of the reference genome). For the most part, this variation is not harmful and makes us distinct individuals, but some variants have been linked to diseases and health-related traits. The presence of some disease-causing variants means a high degree of certainty that the person with the variant will develop the disease. This is true for so-called Mendelian diseases. For other disease-causing variants, the relationship with disease is complex and the variants not very predictive of disease. Establishing the relationship between a genetic variant and disease is accomplished through different research methods. Mendelian and complex diseases differ in terms of the location of disease-causing variants, their frequency in the population, their penetrance, and their utility as diagnostic/predisposition tests.

MENDELIAN GENETIC DISORDERS

Mendelian genetic disorders are individually rare, but in aggregate are present in about 2–3% of all newborns, although disease may not be manifest for years to decades, or ever. They are characterized by a clear pattern of inheritance, typically autosomal dominant, autosomal recessive, or X-linked.

Modes of inheritance

Autosomal dominant

A disease-causing variant in one of the two copies of a gene is sufficient to cause disease. Typical inheritance is from one affected parent who passes the variant to 50% of his or her offspring (Fig. A3-1). These tend to be diseases that occur in adulthood. Both sexes are affected equally. Some common examples include familial hypercholesterolemia (1 in 200), hereditary breast and ovarian cancer (1 in 400), and Lynch syndrome (1 in 400).

Autosomal recessive

Autosomal recessive diseases are the result of two unaffected parents who are each carriers of a mutation in one copy of the gene, and disease results when their child inherits both abnormal copies (Fig. A3-2). These may be two copies of the same variant (homozygote) or two different variants (compound heterozygote). Individuals with only one copy of a disease-causing variant

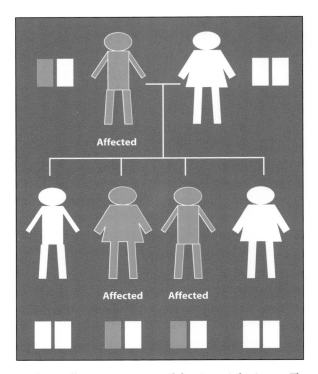

Figure A3-1. **Pedigree illustrating autosomal dominant inheritance.** The most common situation is one affected parent carrying the disease mutation and passing it on to half of their offspring, who also become affected by the disease.

are carriers, but will not develop the disease. When two carriers reproduce, one quarter of their offspring are expected to inherit both disease-causing variants and will manifest the disease, one quarter of offspring inherit two normal copies of the gene, and half will inherit just one and be carriers. Recessive diseases affect both sexes equally and are more prevalent in consanguineous populations. Carrier rates are highest in the United States for sickle cell anemia (1 in 12 African-Americans)[1], cystic fibrosis (1 in 29 Caucasian Americans)[2], and Tay–Sachs (1 in 27 Ashkenazi Jews)[3], although the incidence of these diseases has dropped due to effective genetic screening programs.

Contrary to conventional wisdom, carriers of one copy of a disease-causing variant for a recessive trait are not always unaffected. Some examples: carriers of a Gaucher disease variant are at increased risk of Parkinson disease[4]; carriers of a cystic fibrosis variant are at increased risk of pancreatitis and other disorders[5]; Carriers of a sickle cell anemia variant are at increased risk of exertional rhabdomyolysis and other disorders[6].

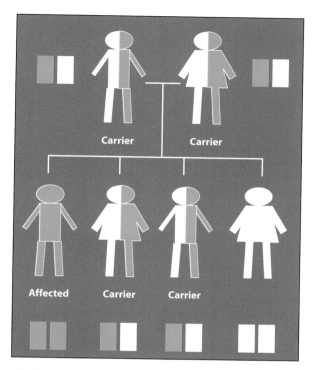

Figure A3-2. Pedigree illustrating autosomal recessive inheritance. The most common situation is two unaffected parents, each carrying a single disease mutation that is passed on to half of their offspring. By chance, 25% of those offspring will inherit both disease mutations and become affected.

X-linked

X-linked inheritance is a special case. Males have only one X chromosome, while females have two. A variant on the X chromosome in a male affects his only copy, which is sufficient to cause disease (it behaves in a dominant fashion). In females, who have two X chromosomes, it behaves more like a recessive where carriers of a single mutation are unaffected. This explains why X-linked traits are more common in males than females. This situation can become even more complicated since one X chromosome, chosen at random, is inactivated, in females. Sometimes because of different patterns of X inactivation in different tissues, female carriers may be symptomatic. Examples of diseases where female carriers of X-linked mutations can frequently be affected (though not necessarily to the same degree as males) include fragile X, Fabry disease, and X-linked adrenoleukodystrophy.

Oddly, some X-linked diseases present only in females. This is usually because the disorder is lethal at an embryonic stage in males. An example is Rett syndrome, caused by mutations in *MECP2*.

Mitochondrial

The cell's powerhouses, the mitochondria, contain their own very small genome consisting of 37 genes, mostly involved in the respiratory chain. Mutations in mitochondrial genes mostly affect cells and organs that have the highest energy consumption, leading to a wide range of disorders, primarily affecting the neuromuscular system. Mitochondrial DNA (mtDNA) is inherited independently of nuclear DNA and only from the mother (the mitochondrial genome is carried in the ova but not the sperm). Mitochondrial disorders due to mutations in the mtDNA can affect males and females equally, but will be transmitted only from the mother. Importantly, most of the proteins present in the mitochondria are encoded in the nuclear genome, meaning that most mitochondrial diseases are not inherited from the mother only and are often recessive.

Because each mitochondrion contains several copies of its genome, and each cell contains many mitochondria, meaning a cell, tissue, or individual can be a mixture of different mitochondrial genomes, a concept termed *heteroplasmy*. Heteroplasmy can cause two individuals with the same change in the mitochondrial genome to have different symptoms determined by which tissues have the abnormal mitochondria, and can cause a woman to pass different amounts of abnormal mitochondrial to her offspring, leading to different symptoms.

De novo

While not inherited, per se, de novo mutations that occur in the sperm or the egg are emerging as an important cause of Mendelian disease in patients with healthy parents. De novo disease-causing mutations can cause dominant or X-linked diseases and can contribute to recessive diseases as well. In all cases, the de novo variant will not be found in either parent, by definition.

Most de novo mutations occur in the egg or sperm that gives rise to a new person and appear in every cell in that person. De novo mutations can also occur after fertilization, in which case the individual will be a mosaic of cells that do and do not harbor a mutation. Mosaicism can range from involving most of the body to only a small fraction of cells.

Methods to discover Mendelian disease genes

Linkage analysis and positional cloning

Prior to the sequencing of the human genome, Mendelian genetic diseases were typically discovered using a laborious method called positional cloning. This method saw its first success in 1986 with the cloning of the gene for X-linked chronic granulomatous disease[7]. Positional cloning takes advantage of multigenerational pedigrees with multiple affected and unaffected individuals analyzed across their genomes for a standard panel of highly variable genetic variants (*markers*). These genetic markers are not thought to be disease-causing variants themselves, but rather, serve to mark,

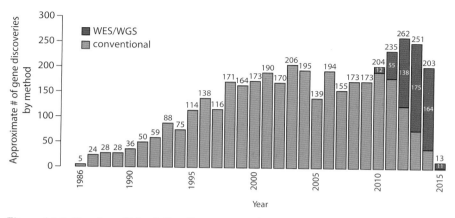

Figure A3-3. **Number of Mendelian disease genes discovered by year.** The number of Mendelian disease genes discovered per year has grown, as has the relative proportion of those discoveries made using next-generation sequencing. (Reproduced with permission from Chong JX, Buckingham KJ, Jhangiani SN, et al: The Genetic Basis of Mendelian Phenotypes: Discoveries, Challenges, and Opportunities, Am J Hum Genet. 2015 Aug 6;97(2):199-215).

or indicate, specific locations in the genome. Linkage analysis involves examining each of these genetic markers to see how well presence of specific marker alleles cosegregate with (i.e., travel with) the disease in the family. Complete cosegregation occurs when the marker allele is present in all affected individuals and absent in all unaffected individuals. The degree to which cosegregation occurs can be statistically measured with a statistic called an LOD score. Genetic markers that exhibit high LOD scores are said to be linked to the disease (more technically, they are linked to the gene underlying the disease). Linkage analysis narrows down the location of a disease gene to a chromosomal region, but further genetic analysis is required to narrow the region down even further, and then to identify candidate genes in that region and confirm their role in disease.

Whole-genome/exome sequencing

The ability to sequence human genomes relatively quickly and cheaply has revolutionized the discovery of Mendelian disease genes. Since 2009, next-generation sequencing has led to a dramatic rise in the number of novel disease-causing genes discovered (Fig. A3-3). The most common approach involves sequencing the whole genomes or exomes of a trio, including an affected individual and his or her parents. A series of data filtering steps based on mutation type, allele frequency, and mode of inheritance narrows down the list of possible candidate genes. These genes are reviewed in depth using information from public databases and the scientific literature to identify the most plausible candidate.

Characteristics of genetic variants associated with Mendelian diseases

Of the approximately 8000 Mendelian traits reported in the Online Mendelian Inheritance in Man (OMIM) database (http://www.ncbi.nlm.nih.gov/omim), the underlying gene is known for over half of them. Sixteen percent of genes in the human genome (3038) are known to underlie a Mendelian trait.[1]

Rare, protein-coding variants

Most genetic variants associated with Mendelian diseases are very rare (<0.1% population allele frequency) protein-altering changes in the coding region of the gene (e.g., truncating mutations, splice site variants, or missense changes), and most (but certainly not all) of these changes cause the gene to not function or function poorly. Less commonly, rare protein-coding variants cause a gene to have extra or new function(s) and these are referred to as gain of function mutations.

Allelic heterogeneity

For a given Mendelian disease gene, there may be more than one variant that can lead to the disease. In some cases, there is one predominant disease-causing variant found in most individuals, and a long tail of rare variants in the gene that round out the population of pathogenic variants. For example, the cystic fibrosis gene, *CFTR*, has one predominant allele, delta F508, found in 85% of cases, but hundreds of additional rare pathogenic variants that also cause cystic fibrosis have been described in the human population.

High penetrance

Mendelian diseases are characterized by having a high penetrance, or probability of developing disease in the presence of a pathogenic variant. However, exceptions to this rule are becoming more evident as more healthy individuals are having their genomes sequenced.

COMPLEX DISEASES

Most diseases are complex, the result of the interplay between genes and environment. Complexity arises from the way that disease is defined, typically based on clinical signs and symptoms or biochemical features, crude measures that might not capture the root molecular cause. Any one clinically defined disease may have forms that are primarily sporadic (environmental in cause), and other forms that are primarily due to inherited gene variants and still others that are due to the interplay of genes and environment. Take leukemia

---

[1] Stats and figure from Centers for Mendelian Genomics: http://www.mendelian.org/about-mendelian-conditions.

for example, where there are rare Mendelian forms due to inherited germline mutations in *TP53* (e.g., Li–Fraumeni syndrome.) There are also sporadic or environmental forms, like the leukemia that developed in atomic bomb survivors exposed to radiation. However, most leukemia is probably due to the cumulative effects of common genetic variants, each individually conferring only a modest increased risk, along with environmental factors. On the clinical level, nongenetic forms of the disease are indistinguishable from genetic forms, making it difficult to discern clear Mendelian inheritance patterns.

Methods to discover genes underlying common, complex diseases

Complex disease gene discovery is typically carried out among large cohorts of subjects that have been characterized with respect to their disease status (affected or unaffected). Subjects with the disease are compared to those without, with respect to the presence of genetic variation. Statistical tests of association are performed to see if the frequency of a genetic variant is different between the two groups. The significance of that association is expressed as a *p* value, and the strength measured in terms of an odds ratio or relative risk.

How does one select which genetic variants to test in an association study? Earlier attempts to identify the genetic basis of complex diseases relied on candidate gene studies, where individual genes likely to play a role in the disease were queried for genetic variation that might be associated with disease. In the early 2000s, genome-wide association studies (GWAS) were introduced as an unbiased way to query the entire genome. By testing hundreds of thousands of variants located throughout the genome, and relying on inherent correlation between variants (linkage disequilibrium), researchers could pinpoint a much smaller region of the genome that might harbor a disease gene. Results of GWAS are often visualized using a Manhattan plot depicting the most statistically significant findings as peaks in a skyline (Fig. A3-4). The type of variation analyzed in these studies is common single nucleotide variants, also called SNPs (single nucleotide polymorphisms). GWAS have dominated the research landscape, identifying dozens of robust associations across myriad diseases and traits. A catalogue of SNPs significantly associated with diseases from GWAS studies is maintained by the NHGRI-EBI (http://www.ebi.ac.uk/gwas/).

Characteristics of complex disease genes

Common noncoding variants

The vast majority (about 90%) of the genetic variants underlying complex diseases are common variants (population allele frequency >5%) located in the noncoding region of the genome (introns and intergenic regions). These variants are concentrated in regulatory regions, suggesting that they impact disease via altering the expression of genes, rather than altering the protein sequence[8].

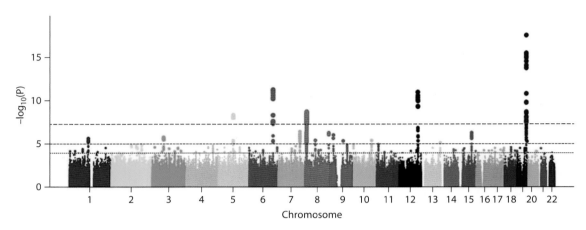

Figure A3-4. Manhattan plot depicting several strongly associated variants from a genome-wide association study (Reproduced with permission from Ikram MK, Sim X, Jensen RA, et al: Four novel Loci (19q13, 6q24, 12q24, and 5q14) influence the microcirculation in vivo, *PLoS Genet.* 2010 Oct 28;6(10):e1001184).

Low penetrance

For most common complex diseases, the penetrance of variants associated with the disease is low. The average effect size for a common variant is about a 1.18-fold increased odds of disease (Fig. A3-5). This is a very modest effect, making these variants individually uninformative as diagnostic/predisposition tests.

CHARACTERISTICS COMMON TO BOTH MENDELIAN AND COMMON COMPLEX DISEASES

Genetic heterogeneity

Both Mendelian and common complex diseases can exhibit genetic heterogeneity, where deleterious mutations in any one of a number of genes may lead to the same disease. For example, dozens of genes have been implicated

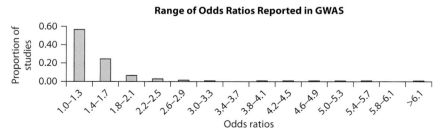

Figure A3-5. Average effect size (in terms of odds ratio) of variants associated with diseases/traits in genome-wide association studies.

in Mendelian forms of nonsyndromic hearing impairment (http://www.ncbi
.nlm.nih.gov/books/NBK1434/). For common diseases, GWAS studies typically reveal dozens of genomic regions associated with the disease (https://
www.ebi.ac.uk/gwas/).

Pleiotropy

Pleiotropy refers to the situation where a single genetic factor influences multiple seemingly distinct traits. Pleiotropy can occur at the level of the gene
(i.e., different variants in the same gene are associated with more than one
trait) or at the level of the variant (i.e., same variant is associated with more
than one trait). About a quarter of known Mendelian disease genes cause two
or more different traits (http://www.mendelian.org/about-mendelian-condi-
tions). Inherited cancer genes are increasingly shown to predispose individuals to more than one type of cancer (see Chapter 7). Complex diseases also
show evidence of pleiotropic effects, especially across different psychiatric
diseases and autoimmune diseases[9]. Pleiotropy is something health care
providers should be aware of as genetic testing for one disease may inform
risk of another.

EVALUATING DISEASE-CAUSING VARIANTS
FOR DIAGNOSTIC/PREDISPOSITION TESTING

The finding of linkage or association of a genetic variant with a disease does
not always mean that the variant will be a clinically valid predictor of disease.
In order to make the jump from research to clinical application, the evidence
supporting that relationship must be evaluated in terms of the robustness,
generalizability, and predictive value of the genetic variant.

How robust is the association?

Robustness of a genetic association in a given research study can be
quantified in terms of statistical significance. Generally, the threshold
for declaring significance of an association found for a complex disease
through GWAS is $p<10^{-8}$, a cutoff that considers multiple testing across
a million variants. In addition to a statistically significant finding in a
single study, the association should be reproducible in a second, separate
population.

For Mendelian disease, the cosegregation of the specific allele with
disease in multiple independent families with the same condition provides evidence of robust linkage. The strength of the evidence ranges from
supporting to strong, depending on the number of independent families
and the strength of linkage of the disease and variant. In addition, genes
implicated in disease are usually required to have supporting evidence
from functional studies demonstrating an effect of the variant on downstream protein structure and/or function.

How generalizable is the association?

Most GWAS are carried out in European populations and the relationship between these variants and disease in other ethnic groups may not have been studied. Some associations are found for different subsets of disease as well, such as early-onset forms, and may not generalize to later-onset disease. Reviewing the primary studies where the associations were found will give the reader a sense of the generalizability.

How predictive is the genetic variant of disease?

The predictive value, or penetrance, of a genetic association describes the strength of the association. This measure of effect is generally calculated from research studies that may be biased or inappropriately designed for producing such estimates. Ideally, the predictive value of test will be determined from prospective studies representative of the population(s) that the test will be applied to. Short of that, one must recognize that risk estimates derived from retrospective research studies (especially case-control studies) may not be accurate.

Penetrance estimates for Mendelian disease gene variants also tend to be biased. Historically they have been calculated from within families with the disease in question. As more and more ostensibly healthy individuals have been sequenced, we are finding individuals carrying these high penetrance variants who don't have the disease, suggesting that earlier penetrance estimates are generally overestimated[10]. Still, penetrance for classic Mendelian disease is still much higher than that for common, complex conditions.

RESOURCES

Online Mendelian Inheritance in Man (OMIM) (http://www.ncbi.nlm.nih.gov/omim)

OMIM is a comprehensive, authoritative compendium of human genes and genetic traits that is freely available and updated daily.

GeneReviews (www.genereviews.org)

An online database containing standardized peer-reviewed articles that describe specific heritable diseases.

Catalog of published genome-wide association studies (GWAS) (https://www.ebi.ac.uk/gwas/)

The GWAS catalog is a searchable, manually curated collection of all published GWAS with significant trait associations.

REFERENCES

1. Lorey FW, Arnopp J, Cunningham GC. Distribution of hemoglobinopathy variants by ethnicity in a multiethnic state. *Genet Epidemiol.* 1996;13:501-512.
2. Strom CM, Crossley B, Buller-Buerkle A, et al. Cystic fibrosis testing 8 years on: lessons learned from carrier screening and sequencing analysis. *Genet Med.* 2011;13:166-172.

3. Scott SA, Edelmann L, Liu L, Luo M, Desnick RJ, Kornreich R. Experience with carrier screening and prenatal diagnosis for 16 Ashkenazi Jewish genetic diseases. *Hum Mutat.* 2010;31:1240-1250.

4. Mitsui J, Mizuta I, Toyoda A, et al. Mutations for Gaucher disease confer high susceptibility to Parkinson disease. *Arch Neurol.* 2009;66:571-576.

5. Noone PG, Zhou Z, Silverman LM, Jowell PS, Knowles MR, Cohn JA. Cystic fibrosis gene mutations and pancreatitis risk: relation to epithelial ion transport and trypsin inhibitor gene mutations. *Gastroenterology.* 2001;121:1310-1319.

6. Tsaras G, Owusu-Ansah A, Boateng FO, Amoateng-Adjepong Y. Complications associated with sickle cell trait: a brief narrative review. *Am J Med.* 2009;122:507-512.

7. Royer-Pokora B, Kunkel LM, Monaco AP, et al. Cloning the gene for the inherited disorder chronic granulomatous disease on the basis of its chromosomal location. *Cold Spring Harb Symp Quant Biol.* 1986;51(pt 1):177-183.

8. Maurano MT, Humbert R, Rynes E, et al. Systematic localization of common disease-associated variation in regulatory DNA. *Science.* 2012;337:1190-1195.

9. Solovieff N, Cotsapas C, Lee PH, Purcell SM, Smoller JW. Pleiotropy in complex traits: challenges and strategies. *Nat Rev Genet.* 2013;14:483-495.

10. Van Driest SL, Wells QS, Stallings S, et al. Association of arrhythmia-related genetic variants with phenotypes documented in electronic medical records. *JAMA.* 2016;315:47-57.

Family History

Family history is a risk factor for many common diseases, capturing both shared genetic variation and shared environment between family members. Because our understanding of genetic risk factors for common diseases is incomplete, family history remains an important component of any medical assessment. A family history of a common disease is usually associated with a two to threefold increased risk of disease in bloodline family relatives. To put this in context, this risk is much higher than for most known individual genetic variants for common diseases (average increased risk for variants discovered to date are about 1.18-fold).

GENETIC AND FAMILIAL ARE NOT SYNONYMOUS

Positive family history, but not genetic

A positive family history of disease does not always mean there is an inherited genetic basis. Family history may reflect shared environment (e.g., exposure of siblings to second-hand smoke). Family history may also reflect chance. For example, cardiovascular disease is the leading cause of death in the United States, where one in three adults have at least one type. Therefore, it would not be surprising to find a positive family history in most cases.

Genetic, with no family history

The absence of a family history does not rule out a genetic basis of disease. Depending on the mode of inheritance and genetic background, a person can inherit a variant and not develop disease, and thus would not contribute to a family history. For example, recessive diseases require two gene variants. X-linked diseases usually require two gene variants in females. De novo variants are not inherited at all, but acquired during the formation of the gametes (though the patient can then pass them to his children). In addition, genetic background may affect penetrance, such as in breast cancer where inherited variants show reduced penetrance for breast cancer in males.

INTERPRETING A FAMILY HISTORY

When capturing family history of disease, it is important to consider the type of relative as well as age of onset and other unusual aspects of disease (Fig. A4-1). Some key points to remember include the following:

- A disease clearly segregating in multiple individuals on either the maternal or paternal side is more significant than having a single affected

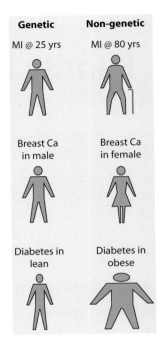

Figure A4-1. **Age of onset and other unusual cases of disease may lend clues to a disease having a genetic etiology.** MI, myocardial infarction; Ca, cancer.

family member on both sides of the family, particularly for common diseases.

- A history of the disease in first-degree family members (parents, siblings, children) is more significant than in distant relatives.
- Early age of onset, especially for a typically later-onset disease, is more significant than later-onset disease (e.g., myocardial infarction in a 25-year-old, vs. an 80-year-old).
- A disease manifesting in the less often affected sex is more likely to be genetic (e.g., breast cancer in a male).
- A disease in the absence of known risk factors is more likely to be genetic (e.g., diabetes in lean vs. overweight individuals).

TIPS FOR COLLECTING A FAMILY HISTORY

Collecting a full family history can be time consuming and beyond the scope of many clinical encounters. Nevertheless, a one-time investment can lay the groundwork for years of precision medicine without sequencing a single nucleotide of DNA! Many electronic health records (EHR) include a mechanism to enter a family history that can be saved and imported into future notes and shared with other providers, though the sophistication of current EHR incorporation of family history has room to evolve. We encourage physicians and other health care practitioners to make collecting a family history a part of establishing a relationship with every new patient.

- If time allows, start with the patient, ask about his or her children (if age-appropriate), then siblings and the sibling's children, then parents, the parents' siblings (uncles and aunts), then their children, then their grandparents. Sometimes it is even worth discussing great uncles and aunts.

- For pediatric patients, it is important to specifically ask about childhood diseases in the family that are likely to have a hereditary component. These include any birth defects, stillbirths or early/sudden deaths, seizures, developmental delay, autism, congenital heart disease, or a parent with recurrent (three or more) miscarriages.

- Don't forget to clarify if siblings are full or half siblings, and if half, which parent is in common.

- If a rare disease is suspected, simply ask if the patient's parents might be related. It may seem unusual in some societies but is an important means to sway the differential diagnosis toward recessive disorders. Consanguinity is common in many cultures and should not be seen as a source of shame.

- Asking about the ethnic/ancestral background of both parents is also important, as many heritable conditions are more common in different parts of the world.

To facilitate collection of family history, patients may be directed to use any of a number of free electronic family history tools described below in the Resources section. These web-based tools allow patients to enter and store their family history, print it out, and share it with others.

ACTIONABILITY OF FAMILY HISTORY

A strong positive family history can indicate risk reduction measures like increased surveillance (e.g., more frequent or earlier colonoscopies in the presence of a family history of colon cancer). Family history may also be an indication for genetic testing, which in turn may lead to prophylactic treatments (e.g., mastectomy or tamoxifen in the case of inherited breast cancer variants). Table A4-1 lists conditions for which there are evidence-based guidelines supporting collection of family history in clinical practice.

Table A4-1. Adult conditions with strong, evidence-based support for capturing family history.

Condition (family history of....)	Utility of family history	Evidence sources
Breast/ovarian or other BRCA-related cancers	Counseling for BRCA genetic testing	USPSTF (2013) NCCN Guideline (2013) NCCN Task Force (2011)
Early-onset cardiovascular disease	Cholesterol screening	USPSTF (2008)
Hip fracture (paternal history)	Osteoporosis screening in women	USPSTF (2011)
Hemochromatosis (sibling history)	Counseling for genetic testing	USPSTF (2006)

Reproduced with permission from the US CDC Office of Public Health Genomics.

RESOURCES

My Family Health Portrait (familyhistory.hhs.gov/FHH/html/index.html)

Interactive web-based tool from the U.S. Surgeon General and the U.S. Centers for Disease Control and Prevention. Collects and stores information on family health history, draws pedigree, and reports risk. Can be modified and printed.

Family History Tool (www.invitae.com/en/familyhistory/)

Web and iPad-based tool from InVitae that allows creation of a detailed and comprehensive digital record of a patient's pedigree, as well as risk assessment. Can be modified, printed, and shared electronically. Secure data storage.

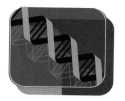

Selecting and Ordering a Lab Test

HOW TO FIND A TESTING LABORATORY

When selecting a laboratory to provide genomic testing for your specific needs, there are many choices to consider. There are hospital and academic laboratories, large reference laboratories, and boutique companies that may all offer similar tests. For clinical testing in the United States, be sure to select a laboratory certified through the Clinical Laboratory Improvement Amendments of 1988 (CLIA).

Several websites offer searchable databases to assist in finding a laboratory and test. We do not endorse a particular site, but the following are non-exhaustive suggestions.

Genetic Testing Registry (GTR) (http://www.ncbi.nlm.nih.gov/gtr/)

This is the official U.S. government website for genetic testing, hosted by the U.S. National Institutes of Health (NIH). It provides more clinical information related to a given gene and condition than other sites, which can be particularly useful for tests sent infrequently or for rare diseases. Filters can also be applied here to narrow by laboratory location, CLIA certification, state licensure, New York State Clinical Laboratory Evaluation Program (CLEP), test methods, specimen type, etc. It is integrated with professional practice guidelines, *GeneReviews*, consumer resources for patients, ClinicalTrials .gov, and all major genetics authorities such as Online Mendelian Inheritance in Man (OMIM) and Orphanet. The advanced test search enables tailored queries such as panel size, specific genes and conditions, pharmacogenetics, prenatal testing, etc. This resource currently has 32,000 clinical and research tests for Mendelian disorders, drug response, and cancer (germline and somatic).

GeneTests (genetests.org)

This site provides labs that perform given gene tests or panels around the world, with the ability to filter based on sequencing method, location, and single gene versus panel. It does not allow filtering by state (could be helpful for insurance reasons), and does not always make it easy to compare gene panels directly to each other. This is a good resource for rare disease genes, or to get a complete list of which labs cover a particular gene of interest. It currently has 55,000 tests.

NextGxDx (nextGxDx.com)

This site is more focused on the United States and is user-friendly for comparing larger panels in terms of which genes are on the panel, price, and other factors. By registering, some tests can be ordered and followed through the site. It currently has 60,000 tests.

Eurogentests (eurogentest.org)

An excellent resource in Europe, which in addition to laboratory and test information provides a wealth of gene and disease information as well (similar to OMIM).

HOW TO SELECT A TEST

There are many clinical diagnostic laboratories (both commercial and academic) around the world that offer a broad range of tests, but little evidence to support the use of one laboratory over another. For simple tests (e.g., targeted genotyping in single genes), cost and turnaround time are probably the most relevant considerations. Local or very large companies are more likely to contract with local insurance. Increasingly, diagnostic laboratories are offering next-generation sequencing gene panels instead of—or in addition to—single-gene analysis. This reflects the reality that many diseases can be caused by changes in more than one gene (genetic heterogeneity). For gene panels, there are a number of factors to consider when choosing a test including the size and gene content of the panel, the method(s) of variant detection, their level of experience interpreting and classifying variants and the resulting rates of variants of uncertain significance (VUS), and the practices and policies of the laboratory around reclassification of variants as more information becomes available. In GTR, labs report their policy about VUS interpretation, recontact, and testing family members on the test interpretation tab (Fig. A5-1).

Gene panel size and content

Gene panels for a given condition may be large or small and the specific genes included on the panel may vary by test provider. Costs may vary according to the number of genes on a panel as well, with larger panels generally being more expensive than smaller ones. In general, smaller panels usually include only high-penetrance genes that are a major cause of the disease, with evidence for each gene supported by guidelines (Fig. A5-2). An example for breast cancer would be a panel testing only the genes *BRCA1* and *BRCA2*. Slightly larger panels may include the most common genes as well as others with only moderate penetrance, greater rarity, and/or less evidence supporting their involvement in the disease in question. An example might be an infantile epilepsy panel which includes the most common genes but also some that that are very rare or for which epilepsy is possible—but not

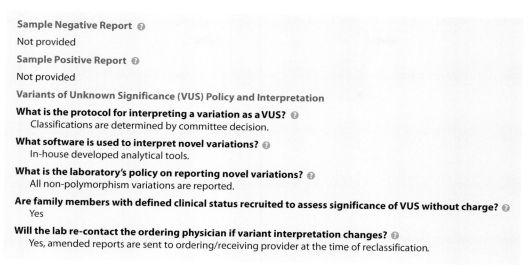

Sample Negative Report @

Not provided

Sample Positive Report @

Not provided

Variants of Unknown Significance (VUS) Policy and Interpretation

What is the protocol for interpreting a variation as a VUS? @
  Classifications are determined by committee decision.

What software is used to interpret novel variations? @
  In-house developed analytical tools.

What is the laboratory's policy on reporting novel variations? @
  All non-polymorphism variations are reported.

Are family members with defined clinical status recruited to assess significance of VUS without charge? @
  Yes

Will the lab re-contact the ordering physician if variant interpretation changes? @
  Yes, amended reports are sent to ordering/receiving provider at the time of reclassification.

Figure A5-1. Sample lab report from the Genetic Testing Registry where they show their policy about VUS interpretation, recontact, and testing family members on the test interpretation tab (Reproduced with permission from the National Institutes of Health, Genetic Testing Registry).

typical—presentation. Even larger panels include many genes that are supported by much less evidence and with unknown penetrance, frequency, and often only rarely associated with the patient's symptoms. Insurance coverage may become more difficult to secure as panels become larger, less focused, and more expensive.

A benefit of ordering larger panels is that the diagnostic yield is improved. A patient who tests negative for the most common hereditary breast cancer genes, *BRCA1* and *BRCA2*, may harbor one of the less common causes of hereditary breast cancer. If the genetic etiology is due to a less common genetic cause, then the answer may be delivered more expeditiously by starting with a larger panel than by sequentially ordering larger and larger panels. The drawback of larger panels is that the results may be less certain. This stems from two factors. The first is that because the broader set of genes is typically less well studied, the interpretation of variants found in these genes (i.e., establishing whether they are pathogenic or not) is more difficult, leading to a higher rate of VUS. These VUS are variants for which there is insufficient evidence to determine if they are disease causing or harmless. The challenge is that discovering such a variant may lead to detrimental and unnecessary testing, screening, or anxiety. In patients who are symptomatic and need a diagnosis, the tolerance for these uncertain variants is higher than in healthy individuals, from whom more caution is warranted. Some companies, for some tests, don't report VUS, or give the option not to have them reported. *Discussing the potential to discover uncertain variants is critical to pretest counseling.*

	Penetrance	Evidence	Attributable %
1	Mod-High	Guidelines	Major cause
2	Mod	Mod	?
3	Unknown	Little	Minor cause

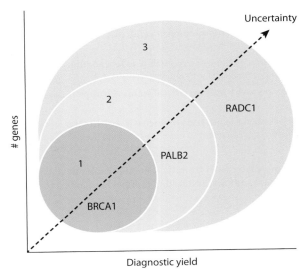

Figure A5-2. Illustration of how the diagnostic yield changes as the size of the gene panel (number of genes) increases. The general characteristics of panels of various sizes with respect to penetrance, evidence, and attributable fraction of the genes on the panel are shown in the table. Examples of category 1, 2, and 3 breast cancer genes are shown.

   The second factor leading to uncertainty of results from expanded panels stems from the unknown penetrance of some of these genes. In other words, it's not clear what the risk of developing cancer (or any condition) is in a person who harbors a pathogenic variant. Even if a variant damages a gene, that observation may not directly translate into a disease for the patient.

   At the end of the day, how narrow or broad to test (i.e., few or many genes at once) depends on the clinical judgment of the ordering physician.

Methods of variant detection

Many laboratories are using next-generation sequencing-based technologies for variant detection, but these may not be able to detect certain types of variants relevant to the disease. The method of detection should match the types of variants likely to cause the disease. Many diseases can be caused by small deletions or duplications within a gene that are invisible to some types of sequencing assays. Detecting such mutations often requires a separate analysis such as del/dup. *If a mutation in a gene is suspected and yet no mutation is detected, the first question a geneticist will ask is "did you get del/dup?"* Some testing laboratories perform this as part of the standard test for a given gene, while for others it must be ordered separately. Particularly in cases where obtaining insurance authorization is difficult, it might be preferable to use a laboratory that performs both tests simultaneously.

Experience with variant interpretation/classification

For genes that can have many and/or complex mutations (e.g., *BRCA1*), one should consider the size of the laboratory's database. This is because laboratories maintain databases of the pathogenicity of variants, and the larger the database, the more likely the lab can provide an accurate and complete interpretation of any detected variants. Many genetics professionals[1] (including the authors of this text) believe that all diagnostic labs should submit all variants and de-identified clinical data to public databases (see www.free-the-data.org), but such open access is not legally required and some diagnostic companies maintain proprietary databases. In some cases (particularly Myriad Genetic Laboratories, Inc. with regard to *BRCA1* and *BRCA2* testing) the proprietary databases may be superior to those that are publically available, but sending testing to these companies restricts public access to new variants.

Reclassification of variants

Over time, as more scientific evidence is accumulated, the status of a VUS may change. Practices around variant reclassification vary by testing laboratory in terms of whether and how often they routinely review new evidence in an attempt to reclassify, and if/how reclassified variants are reported to the ordering physician. Check with the laboratory's policy regarding how often they reevaluate variants and how reclassifications are communicated to the customer.

Gene coverage

Many large gene panels use next-generation technology, which loses about 5–10% of sequence coverage due to technical limitations. Some labs fill in these gaps with highly reliable Sanger sequencing (termed Sanger backfill) while others do not. When thorough analysis of specific genes is desired the ordering physician should consider a more focused panel or one that completes areas of low coverage with Sanger sequencing.

For specialty panels (e.g., prenatal carrier panels, pharmacogenomics panels), please see the relevant chapter.

[1] http://nsgc.org/p/bl/et/blogid=47&blogaid=330
http://www.ama-assn.org/ama/pub/news/news/2013/2013-06-18-new-ama-policies-annual-meeting.page

HOW TO ORDER A TEST

Many clinicians find ordering genetic testing to be daunting. Like any clinical skill there are key concepts to ensure that the correct test is done for the correct patient, but there is no reason a priori that a nongeneticist practitioner cannot send genetic testing for his or her own patients. The following covers the key points to empower physicians and other providers to send genetic testing when referral to a specialist is difficult, might delay care, or may not be necessary. See Appendix 7 for issues surrounding billing and insurance authorization. Specifics vary by the testing laboratory and the lab obtaining the sample, but the following are generalities that apply in most situations.

- Most tests are done on blood. A few can be done on saliva, buccal samples, or dried blood spots. Blood is almost always collected in an EDTA tube if intended for DNA sequencing. A small number of specialized tests require fibroblasts cultured from a skin biopsy. Prenatal testing is usually done on chorionic villi or amniocytes. Formalin-fixed paraffin-embedded samples are difficult to sequence; obtain fresh frozen samples if sending testing on tissue.

- Fill out the test requisition provided by the testing laboratory, which can usually be found on their website. Often clinical information is requested, and it can be helpful to provide some documentation such as a clinic note. The more complex the test and the more genes being tested, the more the laboratory will want clinical information to help sift through their sequencing results. *For large gene panels or exomes, the quality of results depends significantly on providing quality phenotype information.*

- Most laboratories provide collection details for each test on their website, including the type of tube, amount of blood, and shipping instructions. If the tests will be sent by the provider him/herself, many companies will provide, upon request, a collection kit with necessary tubes, labels, cool packs, etc., often with shipping labels. Hospitals or larger centers may have their own department to package and send-out labs, and this department will generally be familiar with protocols for mailing DNA specimens. If genetic testing will frequently be required, it would behoove a practitioner to identify the individual(s) involved in sending out labs to facilitate a smooth process every time. *If possible, do not ship specimens on Fridays or before holidays, as this frequently delays delivery and can lead to sample degradation.*

- Many hospitals and medical centers can isolate and store DNA until it is sent to a laboratory. When it is difficult to align the timing of a blood draw with actually sending the test, this can be preferable because frozen DNA is stable for years.

- Turnaround times for genetic tests vary widely, but are often four weeks at a minimum for any nonroutine test, and can be several months for multigene tests. Some companies will expedite testing (particularly on

Table A5-1. Major genetic diagnostic laboratories in the United States.

Laboratory	Link
InVitae	https://www.invitae.com/
GeneDx	http://www.genedx.com/
Ambry Genetics	http://www.ambrygen.com/
Prevention Genetics	https://www.preventiongenetics.com/
Baylor Miraca Genetics Laboratories	http://bmgl.com/
Fulgent	https://fulgentdiagnostics.com/
Emory Genetics Laboratory	http://geneticslab.emory.edu/
Athena Diagnostics	http://www.athenadiagnostics.com/
Greenwood Genetics	http://www.ggc.org/

fetal samples, but often for any age) for an additional charge that may or may not be covered by insurance. The delay to receive results should be considered when clinical decisions will depend on the result of testing.

• For questions or concerns, most laboratories are eager to sell tests and will have both telephone customer service and local representatives who will assist in escorting samples through the collection, shipping, and analysis process and ensure that paperwork is done correctly.

Major genetic diagnostic laboratories in the United States are listed in Table A5-1. These were selected based on providing a wide range of genetics and genomics services. They are listed in no particular order, and the list is not exhaustive. Specialty labs are listed where appropriate in some other chapters. Carrier screening is discussed in Chapter 1. Cell-free DNA prenatal screening is discussed in Chapter 2. Some metabolic labs are listed in Chapter 4. Some labs offering chromosomal microarrays and exome sequencing are listed in Chapter 5. Some labs offering tumor profiling are listed in Chapter 9.

WHO TO TEST

Before sending genetic testing, it is important to know which individual is the most appropriate to initiate testing. It is not always the patient who asks! A minority of diseases, such as Huntington disease, are caused by a single type of genetic change in a single gene. In such conditions, the presence or absence of the disease can be determined with high confidence in any individual by testing for one change in one gene. However, Huntington disease is an exception, and most diseases can be caused by countless variants anywhere in several to dozens of genes.

For this reason, *the first step is to test the patient or family member most likely to have the disease-causing variant in a gene.* For example, if a healthy woman asks for *BRCA1* and *BRCA2* sequencing because of breast cancer in her sister, it would be optimal to test the sister with cancer first. If the sister with cancer had a mutation in *BRCA1* identified, then the presence or absence of this mutation in the unaffected sister would be interpretable findings in terms of her breast cancer risk. But if the unaffected sister were tested alone, it would be impossible to distinguish between several possibilities: the healthy sister may not have inherited her sister's *BRCA1* mutation, the affected sister's cancer may have been unrelated to *BRCA1*, or the mutation in *BRCA1* may be difficult to identify by standard tests (and the patient may have this mutation despite a negative genetic test).

INFORMED CONSENT = PRETEST COUNSELING

While genetic counseling is sometimes considered to be a specialty of its own, any practitioner who orders genetic tests should consider this counseling as ethically mandatory as any informed consent before, for example, a surgical procedure. Indeed, performing genetic testing infrequently produces definitive results, instead providing complex information that relies on the clinical context, existing literature, and professional experience. All genetic tests demand that the patient be reminded that many genetic conditions are inherited and that the result of any genetic test may be relevant to family members. Beyond this, the level of detail required for proper informed consent varies by the nature of the test being ordered.

- For broader tests that sequence whole genes or analyze chromosomes, several points should be discussed with patients to fully inform them of the benefits and risks associated with testing. The tests fall into two categories, each with distinct points:
  - For tests that that only report interpretable results and not VUS, like most expanded carrier screening panels (see Chapter 1), the patient must be informed that a negative result substantially reduces the risk that they have a mutation in that gene, but some variants may not have been reported and residual risk remains.
  - For diagnostic tests that report all variants, including VUS, much of the frustration that comes with uncovering a VUS can be avoided if the patient was educated about this eventuality before testing was sent. Tests such as NIPS (see Chapter 2) can return uninterpretable or indeterminate results and fall into this category.
  - The same can be said for many metabolic screening tests (see Chapter 4). Because many metabolites are tested simultaneously, it is common for some to be slightly out of the normal range and neither conclusively positive or negative.

- Targeted genotyping tests that seek the presence or absence of a specific variant are essentially yes-or-no tests, so VUS are not an issue. However, the patient should be educated as to the purpose and benefits of the test, as well as the performance characteristics (e.g., how well they predict disease).

For genome-wide tests that sequence many genes (e.g., whole exome or whole genome), patients must be informed that this test might uncover a variant in a gene that affects their health that is totally unrelated to the reason the test was sent, so-called "incidental" or "secondary" findings. A typical example is discovering a *BRCA1* mutation on an exome sent for a child with autism. Another example is discovering cancer in a pregnant woman undergoing noninvasive prenatal screening on cell-free DNA. Patients or their parents can opt out of receiving these secondary findings and this discussion is essential before sending any genome-wide test.

However, importantly, these tests are not intended to identify unrelated disease genes and therefore the lack of a report does not mean the family does not carry a given gene. Some diagnostic labs search for the American College of Medical Genetics and Genomics (ACMG) recommended secondary findings in all samples, while others only look in the proband (the patient) and only check the relatives (usually parents) for variants found in the proband; thus a parent may have a pathogenic allele for an actionable disease, but if the child did not inherited it then that variant may not be reported.

Most genome-wide tests also have the potential to uncover unexpected family relationships, such as consanguinity or false paternity. Patient can often opt out of this information, too, but sometimes it is difficult to avoid disclosing. For example, if a trio exome (a child and both parents) is sent, and the paternal sample is not from the biological father, then determination of the inheritance of variants in the child will be limited and directly reduce the yield of the test.

> **Key Point**
>
> If a family believes they may carry a genetic disease, the absence of detection of this disease on whole-exome (or genome) sequencing sent for unrelated reasons is not evidence that this disease gene is absent in the family. Targeted testing should be pursued if the family wants more definitive information.

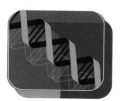

Interpreting the Pathogenicity of Genetic Variants

Next-generation sequencing gene panels for diagnostic or predisposition testing can be expected to uncover genetic variants in every patient tested. However, not all of these variants are disease causing. It is the role of the clinical testing lab to interpret and classify genetic variants as disease causing (pathogenic) or benign. For a health care provider who may order these tests, it is important to understand the rapidly evolving science and art of how these classifications are made.

> **Key Point**
>
> Even a general understanding of the methods used in variant interpretation will give health care providers an appreciation for the limitations of currently available genomic medicine.

VARIANT CLASSIFICATION

There is currently no set standard for classifying variants, but groups like the ClinGen consortium (www.clinicalgenome.org) are working to define standard procedures for classifying and curating sequence variants. The most widely used framework for classifying variants in disease genes is based on an earlier set of guidelines proposed by the American College of Medical Genetics and Genomics (ACMG)[1]. Because classification often occurs in the context of incomplete information, it is rarely definitive, but rather, couched in terms of certainty. The five-tiered ACMG classification (pathogenic, likely pathogenic, uncertain significance (VUS), likely benign, and benign) applies to moderately and highly penetrant disease genes. Low-penetrance disease gene variants, such as those that come from Genome-Wide Association Studies (GWAS), are almost always common variants and are categorized separately as risk factors. The new ACMG guidelines, updated in 2015, provide a much more detailed framework for variant classification[2]. Not all laboratories follow this guideline exactly, nor do they necessarily use the same vocabulary when reporting results. However, most laboratories consider roughly the same evidence in making a determination about variant pathogenicity.

When evaluating a variant, two fundamental considerations are made: first, can the gene containing the variant be plausibly linked to a disease, and second, does the variant affect the function of the gene? All of the following discussion aims at answering these deceptively simple questions.

EVIDENCE USED IN ASSESSMENT OF PATHOGENICITY

Effect of variant on protein structure or function

Any type of variant can be pathogenic, although the likelihood decreases substantially when considering nonprotein-coding variants. Putative loss of function (LOF) variants (stop-gained, stop-lost, frameshift insertion/ deletion, splice site disruptor AG/GT) are the most deleterious and best candidates for pathogenic variants. Missense variants can also be pathogenic, but it's difficult to know if any given missense variant will impact the protein in such a way as to cause disease. Computational algorithms that estimate deleteriousness based on features like conservation and location include programs like PhyloP, Polyphen, SIFT, MutationTaster, and others. These algorithms can best be described as informative but imperfect. Also, variants that occur in mutational hotspots within the gene where other known pathogenic variants cluster, and are of the same type of variant previously associated with the disease, favor pathogenicity.

Allele frequency in others with and without the disease

In the absence of families, presence of the specific variant in multiple independent individuals affected with the same condition and absence in unrelated healthy persons supports pathogenicity. Conversely, if a variant is thought to have high penetrance, identifying an unaffected individual with the same variant provides evidence against pathogenicity. *Rare* variants, those having a frequency in the population less than expected based on the disease frequency, allelic heterogeneity, and mode of inheritance, are more likely pathogenic. For example, the risk of breast cancer in the population is about 11%, but only 5–10% of breast cancer is thought to be inherited. Moreover, there are hundreds of variants that can lead to breast cancer. Therefore, any single variant underlying breast cancer should have an allele frequency less than 1%.

Human genetic linkage/cosegregation studies

Human genetic evidence is derived from family or population-based (unrelated individuals) studies, where observed coinheritance or correlation of a variant with a disease phenotype is inferred from statistical linkage (for family studies) or association (for population studies). This is the most direct and important evidence for pathogenicity of a variant, but also the most difficult to obtain. Sometimes a variant can be reclassified as this type of data accumulates.

In vivo/in vitro studies of variant function

Various laboratory in vivo, ex vivo, or in vitro experiments may support pathogenicity of a variant. The evidence is strongest when the experiment involves an observable phenotype that is consistent with the condition under investigation. Examples of these types of studies include the use of cell-based assays or animal models where the variant can be shown to disrupt the gene or alter a relevant phenotype or where repair of the variant can rescue a phenotype. Many metabolic enzymes have clinically available activity assays that can be used to assess the impact of a variant. Otherwise, most functional gene studies are considered research.

Previous classification as pathogenic

Increasingly, known variants are deposited into locus-specific databases and large variant repositories like the commercially available Human Gene Mutation Database (HGMD®)[3] and ClinVar[4], the largest publicly available repository. ClinVar includes all variants from OMIM, some locus-specific databases, as well as variants submitted by individual testing labs. Submitters to ClinVar often provide a classification of the variant, according to their interpretation. These classifications are mapped onto the ACMG framework (pathogenic, likely pathogenic, VUS, likely benign, benign) for consistency. At present, approximately three-quarters of ClinVar variants are preclassified, but some have multiple conflicting classifications. ClinVar records may or may not contain the supporting evidence to back up their classifications, but sometimes contain links to PubMed articles.

WEIGHING THE EVIDENCE

These lines of evidence, and others, may be combined or weighed differently by individual testing laboratories. Consequently, it is possible that different labs will offer contradictory classifications of variants. One study found a low rate of concordance when examining potentially pathogenic variants in two arrhythmia genes with a two-lab concordance rate of 33% and three-lab concordance rate of only 10%[5]. Similarly, major discrepancies in classification are found when comparing publicly accessible variant databases[6].

A variant that lacks an evidence base to declare it as pathogenic or benign will fall into a gray zone—a VUS. VUS rates vary from lab to lab. Often, laboratories that have run the most tests are able to classify variants more easily. VUS rates are also lower for genes that are generally well studied and higher for those less well studied.

Because of the degree of uncertainty around variant pathogenicity in many cases, variants found upon testing, without a definitive classification, should be reevaluated periodically. Over time, as more evidence accumulates, classifications should be more definitive.

COMMUNICATING WITH THE PATIENT

It is irresponsible, in our opinion, to express confidence in having achieved a genetic diagnosis or doubt a diagnosis beyond what is warranted by available evidence. Ascribing pathogenicity to a variant may cause the patient to stop seeking a diagnosis, may lead to major reproductive decisions, and may suggest invasive screening or other medical (mis)adventures. Ignoring a variant may delay the patient's diagnosis. Still, a core facet of the practice of medicine is the obligation to make clinical decisions, and paralysis in the face of uncertain evidence is hardly preferable to over- or under-action. Rather, any clinician who utilizes genetic testing must be prepared to:

- Consider the likelihood of identifying uncertain variants, and the potential health implications thereof, *before* ordering a test.
- Counsel patients on the possibility and ramifications of VUS *before* ordering a test.
- Invest the time needed to fully understand the results from the laboratory and how they were derived.
- Communicate with specialists, including genetic counselors, as needed.
- Include and educate the patient in understanding what is and is not known about a variant and the involved gene.
- Weigh the risks and benefits of acting or not acting on a variant.
- Request that the laboratory reanalyze the variant after sufficient time has passed, or educate the patient that reanalysis is possible should they desire it in the future.

RESOURCES

Locus specific database (LSDB) list (http://grenada.lumc.nl/LSDB_list/lsdbs)

List of LSDBs based on various online resources and direct submissions, maintained by Leiden University Medical Center.

Human Gene Mutation Database (HGMD) (http://www.hgmd.org)

The public version of HGMD is freely available to registered users from academic institutions/nonprofit organizations while the subscription version (HGMD Professional) is available to academic, clinical, and commercial users under license via BIOBASE GmbH.

ClinVar (www.ncbi.nlm.nih.gov/clinvar/)

A freely available searchable database from the NCBI of variants and their clinical classifications. The database includes germline and somatic variants of any size, type, or genomic location. Interpretations are submitted by clinical testing laboratories, research laboratories, locus-specific databases, OMIM®, GeneReviews™, UniProt, expert panels, and practice guidelines.

The Significance of Unknown Significance: A Teachable Moment (http://www.medscape.com/viewarticle/865546?src=par_jmbm_stm_mscpedt&faf=1)

A discussion of a lawsuit related to variant interpretation that highlights salient methods and pitfalls in interpreting genetic test results.

REFERENCES

1. Richards CS, Bale S, Bellissimo DB, et al. ACMG recommendations for standards for interpretation and reporting of sequence variations: revisions 2007. *Genet Med.* 2008;10:294-300.
2. Richards S, Aziz N, Bale S, et al. Standards and guidelines for the interpretation of sequence variants: a joint consensus recommendation of the American College of Medical Genetics and Genomics and the Association for Molecular Pathology. *Genet Med.* 2015;17:405-424.
3. Stenson PD, Mort M, Ball EV, Shaw K, Phillips A, Cooper DN. The Human Gene Mutation Database: building a comprehensive mutation repository for clinical and molecular genetics, diagnostic testing and personalized genomic medicine. *Hum Genet.* 2014;133:1-9.
4. Landrum MJ, Lee JM, Benson M, et al. ClinVar: public archive of interpretations of clinically relevant variants. *Nucleic Acids Res.* 2016;44:D862-D868.
5. Van Driest SL, Wells QS, Stallings S, et al. Association of arrhythmia-related genetic variants with phenotypes documented in electronic medical records. *JAMA.* 2016;315:47-57.
6. Vail PJ, Morris B, van Kan A, et al. Comparison of locus-specific databases for BRCA1 and BRCA2 variants reveals disparity in variant classification within and among databases. *J Community Genet.* 2015; 6:351-359.

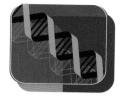

Regulation and Reimbursement

Regulatory and reimbursement decisions for precision medicine tests are based in large part upon a body of evidence around three performance characteristics of the test: analytical validity, clinical validity, and clinical utility. We will first review these concepts and then discuss the current regulatory and reimbursement environment in the United States.

PERFORMANCE CHARACTERISTICS

ANALYTICAL VALIDITY

Analytical validity refers to the accuracy of the laboratory test, that is, how well the assay detects what it is intended to detect. In the case of genetic testing, it refers to how well the testing platform accurately measures and reports a given genetic variant, for example. Analytical validity is usually measured in terms of the test's sensitivity and specificity, which capture information about the likelihood of true versus false positive or true versus false-negative results.

CLINICAL VALIDITY

Clinical validity addresses if the test is clinically meaningful, for example, how well a test can predict a clinical outcome (e.g., disease development, disease progression, or efficacy/toxicity of a drug). These measures are usually derived from statistically robust observational studies. Typical metrics derived from these studies include relative risk, hazard ratios, sensitivity and specificity (sometimes referred to as clinical sensitivity and specificity in this case to distinguish it from analytical sensitivity and specificity discussed above), positive predictive value (PPV), and negative predictive value (NPV) of the test. The strongest evidence comes from synthesizing a body of evidence, as is done for clinical practice guidelines and systematic reviews.

In terms of the measures of effect, the clinical PPV indicates how often someone with a specific genotype will experience the outcome. It is effectively the same as penetrance, a genetic term that denotes the probability that a person who tests positive for the genetic marker will develop the outcomes (disease in this case). Clinical PPV is highly dependent on how common the outcome is. A test for a rare disease or adverse event will never have a high PPV for that outcome. In these cases, NPV may be the more relevant metric. A high NPV usually indicates that most if not all of the people who develop the disease or adverse event will test positive for the specific biomarker. Therefore, a negative test is used to rule out the possible occurrence of the event. This is the case for a genetic test for HLA type and celiac disease. Celiac has a population prevalence of about 1% and virtually all patients with celiac have one of two common HLA variants, DQ2 or DQ8. For this relatively uncommon disorder, this translates into a high NPV, or the ability to rule out celiac in patients who lack these HLA variants.

High clinical PPV is difficult to achieve for common, complex diseases, where the genetic variant associated with the disease is common as well, in large part because the genetics of common diseases is complex and known genetic variants are only a fraction of the entire picture. For rare Mendelian disorders, where the causal genetic variant is also rare, a high penetrance/PPV is more attainable.

CLINICAL UTILITY

In general, clinical utility refers to whether the test will impact health care decisions, lead to measurable improved outcomes, and have a favorable risk/benefit profile.

The exact definition of clinical utility and the amount of evidence required to support it varies by stakeholder[1]. Some stakeholders still insist on randomized controlled clinical trials as the gold standard of demonstrating clinical utility, but this bar may be unrealistic to reach for rare outcomes, leading some to suggest alternative approaches[2].

In summary, the countless possible genetic tests all exist in a framework of highly variable evidence of analytical and clinical validity, and clinical utility, and regulators and payers are left to sort out what should be allowed and what should be reimbursed.

REGULATION OF GENETIC TESTING IN THE UNITED STATES

The current U.S. regulatory landscape for genomic tests is in a state of evolution. Historically, most genomic tests have been classified as laboratory-developed tests (LDTs), offered by a specific laboratory as a service. Although the U.S. Food and Drug Administration (FDA) has had the authority to regulate LDTs, it has chosen not to, exercising its enforcement discretion. Instead, LDTs have been regulated through the Centers for Medicare and Medicaid Services (CMS). CMS ensures that laboratories performing genetic tests comply with the Clinical Laboratory Improvement Amendments of 1988 (CLIA). This certification is primarily concerned with the laboratory's ability to provide analytically valid test results, although it does not evaluate the specific tests per se, but rather, the laboratory environment. Historically, LDTs have *not* been scrutinized or regulated based on their clinical validity or clinical utility.

In 2010, the FDA stated that it intended to begin regulating LDTs, citing concerns over safety and the increasing complexity of some of the new genomic tests.[1] The safety concerns stem from a report of 20 documented cases where patients who underwent testing reportedly experienced harm.[2] This harm resulted from false-positive results, leading to unnecessary treatment or distress, as well as false-negative results, where patients failed to receive treatment for diseases that the test didn't detect. The newly proposed FDA-clearance process for genomic tests will evaluate not only the analytical validity, but the clinical validity of the test too, in an effort to increase the safety of these tests.

The details of these sweeping changes to the regulation of LDTs are still being worked out and are the subject of much controversy and discontent by many in the medical community. In 2014, the FDA announced that it will take a risk-based approach to regulating LDTs that will be phased in over time.[3] Genomic tests will be classified into one of three classes (class I low risk, class II moderate risk, class III high risk) according to their intended use and level of risk they pose to patients if the test results are not accurate (e.g., risk of misdiagnosis or treatment error).

The regulatory controls that will be imposed on tests in these classes is meant to ensure safety and efficacy of these tests. These controls will vary by class, with increasing controls required for tests of increasing risk. High-risk tests, such as those that generate prognostic information linked to therapeutic decision-making, will require the strictest controls, including premarket review. For low-risk tests and tests for rare diseases, on the other hand, the FDA may continue to simply exercise enforcement discretion.

Many stakeholders argue that increased regulation of genomic tests will slow progress in the field and restrict access. Laboratory trade groups have challenged the authority of the FDA to regulate LDTs. At the same time, others point to the proliferation of tests that may not be safely sustainable without some oversight. How these arguments play out will have far reaching implications for the field of precision medicine.

INSURANCE COVERAGE AND REIMBURSEMENT OF GENOMIC TESTS IN THE UNITED STATES

Lack of insurance coverage is a major obstacle for the uptake of novel precision medicine tools in the United States and elsewhere. Health insurance plans look at the test's accuracy (analytical and clinical validity) but also want to know if the test has clinical utility and if it will be cost-effective to cover the test. (Note: neither regulatory pathway for genomic tests—LDT or FDA-approved diagnostic test—requires evidence of clinical utility, which is

---

[1] https://www.federalregister.gov/articles/2010/06/17/2010-14654/oversight-of-laboratory-developed-tests-public-meeting-request-for-comments

[2] http://www.fda.gov/downloads/AboutFDA/ReportsManualsForms/Reports/UCM472777.pdf

[3] http://www.fda.gov/downloads/medicaldevices/deviceregulationandguidance/guidancedocuments/ucm416685.pdf

typically expected for insurance coverage and reimbursement.) Insurers use several sources of data to make decisions about clinical utility, including technology assessments, professional guidelines, FDA clearance, and other payers.

Preauthorization

Many insurance companies require preauthorization for genetic tests, and even when authorized, the copayment or coinsurance can be substantial. At least an estimate of the out-of-pocket cost should be determined before ordering a test to avoid surprise bills. Some diagnostic companies will perform the authorization and out-of-pocket estimate themselves before starting testing, a very useful service if available. Importantly, some diagnostic labs will hold a blood sample until the test is authorized and the patient agrees to the out-of-pocket cost. This approach reduces the risk that a patient will be lost to follow-up while awaiting preauthorization. Always provide the diagnostic company with a copy of the patient's insurance card and, if needed, the letter of authorization.

General coverage patterns

Table A7-1 illustrates how general insurance patterns vary by health plan and are highly complex, variable, and constantly evolving. Verify in each case!

Table A7-1. Insurance patterns by health plan.

Insurance plan	Policy
Medicare	Private insurance companies often look to Medicare, the largest health insurance program in the United States for coverage decisions and then follow suit. Some of the challenges with this practice stem from the fact that Medicare serves an older population (65+). As such, tests in newborns, children, or pregnant women will not be addressed by Medicare, so private insurers need to evaluate those tests on their own. Medicare covers tests that are *reasonable and necessary* for the diagnosis or treatment of illness or injury. Therefore, genomic tests used to diagnose or determine treatment in the presence of signs and symptoms of disease are more likely to be covered by Medicare, but predisposition tests in healthy individuals are not.
PPOs	Generally cover most genetic tests without authorization, but often require the patient to pay the entire deductible and/or substantial coinsurance. Many PPOs have separate in- and out-of-network deductibles, so don't be fooled if a patient has met his or her in-network deductible but the diagnostic lab is out-of-network.
HMOs	Almost always require authorization. Authorization usually depends on the potential to impact management. Unfortunately, many insurers do not consider establishing a diagnosis, clarifying prognosis, or providing reproductive counseling to constitute "management." Prepare a clear letter of medical necessity and expect to file appeals.
Medicaid	Varies by state and often within a state, but in general coverage can be poor, with limited contracted labs and a high bar to obtain insurance authorization. Some states centralize Medicaid, while others give subsidies to privately managed care plans, and each model affects the likelihood of obtaining coverage. Access to testing for Medicaid patients must usually be determined on an individual basis.

Table A7-2. Genetic services categorically addressed in 65 insurer coverage policies (from Graf et al).

Service	Insurers that address service (n)	Insurers that cover, n (%)	Insurers that do not cover, n (%)
Genetic testing (diagnostic)	38	38 (100)	0 (0)
Genetic testing (presymptomatic)	35	31 (89)	4 (11)
Preimplantation genetic diagnosis	28	23 (82)	5 (18)
Genetic counseling	24	24 (100)	0 (0)
Carrier testing (general)	15	12 (80)	3 (20)
Prenatal diagnosis	15	15 (100)	0 (0)
Amniocentesis	12	12 (100)	0 (0)
Direct-to-consumer genetic testing	12	0 (0)	12 (100)
Chorionic villus sampling	11	11 (100)	0 (0)
Recurrent miscarriage genetic evaluation	7	7 (100)	0 (0)
Gene therapy	3	0 (0)	3 (100)
Pharmacogenetic testing	3	3 (100)	0 (0)

Reproduced with permission from Graf MD, Needham DF, Teed N, et al: Genetic testing insurance coverage trends: a review of publicly available policies from the largest US payers, Personalized Medicine 2013 May;10(3):235-243.

A review of health plan genomic testing policies in the United States published in 2013[4] found that for many broad categories of genomic testing, insurance companies had no policies in place (Table A7-2). Among those with policies in place, the coverage was relatively uniform between insurance plans. For example, direct-to-consumer genetic testing was uniformly not covered, while genetic counseling was uniformly covered. Uniform coverage was also found for some specific tests, among those insurers with policies (Table A7-3).

Coverage of next-generation sequencing gene panels

According to research on coverage of next-generation sequencing, reimbursement for disease-specific gene panels using NGS is highly variable and often negotiated on a case-by-case basis[3]. For the purpose of identifying off-label or investigational therapies coverage is generally denied for large gene panels greater than 50 genes (CPT code 81455) because not all of the analytes have proven clinical utility. Some providers opt to use tiered coding (e.g., billing

---

[4] Graf MD, Needham DF, Teed N, Brown T. Genetic testing insurance coverage trends: a review of publicly available policies from the largest US payers. *Pers Med.* 2013;10(3):235–243.

Table A7-3. Genetic tests addressed by at least 10 insurers and uniformly covered (from Graf et al).

Test	Plans addressing (and covering) test, *n*
BRCA1/2 gene sequencing	53
HNPCC/Lynch syndrome gene testing	47
Familial adenomatous polyposis (including attenuated)	46
MSI/IHC colorectal tumor screening	38
KRAS mutation analysis for colorectal cancer	35
First trimester screening	24
Medullary thyroid cancer *RET* gene testing	24
Fragile X syndrome testing	21
Factor V Leiden genetic testing	20
Hemochromatosis genetic testing	19
HIV tropism	19
BRAF (V600E) mutation analysis for melanoma	13
Multiple endocrine neoplasia gene testing	13
HER2 immunohistochemistry	12
HER2 Fish	12
HIV genotyping	12
Celiac disease HLA typing	11

HNPCC, hereditary nonpolyposis colon cancer; IHC, immunohistochemistry; MSI, microsatellite instability (Reproduced with permission from Graf MD, Needham DF, Teed N, et al: Genetic testing insurance coverage trends: a review of publicly available policies from the largest US payers, Personalized Medicine 2013 May;10(3):235-243).

only medically necessary genes on the panel) for reimbursement in this case. Strategies for billing government and private payers and a reviewer of private payer policies are discussed in a recent review. Coverage and reimbursement in this space is evolving.

Coverage of WES/WGS

At the time of writing, Cigna has become the first national health plan to lay out coverage criteria for whole-exome sequencing (WES). The policy says it would cover WES when a patient meets all the criteria on a detailed list.[5] For example, a board-certified geneticist or physician specialist must determine that testing will impact a patient's clinical decisions and outcomes; that the illness is likely due to genetics and not environmental exposures, injury, or infection; that the features of the disease suggest that single-gene testing or panel testing wouldn't be sufficient, and that WES would avoid multiple, invasive workups.

Coding and insurance billing

Once a test receives a positive coverage decision, assignment of a corresponding code enables billing and reimbursement for specific services. Codes for molecular diagnostic tests usually have two components: a laboratory component and a professional services (interpretation) component. Coding and billing for molecular diagnostics remains fluid. The biggest challenge is establishing appropriate compensation for all components of a molecular test, not just the laboratory component, but test interpretation, communication of results/counseling, and follow-up.

Institutional billing is when the practice or medical center must pay for the test directly, and then can seek payment from the patient or his/her insurance. Only accepting institutional billing allows smaller diagnostics companies to avoid the complexity of contracting with countless private insurers around the country. For the practitioner, this practice can ease the process of obtaining genetic testing because the payment is guaranteed up front and testing need not be delayed while seeking authorization, but it does expose the center to the risk that authorization will be denied. Some centers do not permit institutional billing.

Other payment methods

Some companies and hospital/academic laboratories offer patient assistance programs based on need. Make sure to inquire if this is available.

MEDICAL NECESSITY

When seeking to order genetic testing of any kind, it is often necessary to obtain insurance authorization before sending the test (some diagnostics companies will do this themselves with assistance from the ordering physician). Genetic tests can cost >$10,000 and failing to confirm that coverage is adequate places patients at risk for medical bills they may not be able to afford[4]. For in-patient labs, the hospital may have its own internal review process for tests sent out to other labs. In every case, it can be important (and sometimes essential) to provide a letter of medical necessity outlining the rationale for the test. Every insurer is different, and thus only general advice can be provided here.

---

[5] https://cignaforhcp.cigna.com/public/content/pdf/coveragePolicies/medical/mm_0519_coverage positioncriteria_exome_genome_sequence.pdf

In our experience, insurers are singly interested in the potential for a test to *affect management*. The myriad ways that simply having (or ruling out) a diagnosis improves medical care are not obvious to insurers, and one has to paint a clear picture of exactly what decisions will be affected by a test result.

For some tests this is straightforward: "If sequencing shows that the patient's symptoms are explained by Gaucher disease, she will start enzyme replacement therapy." The test-treatment connection is obvious. This becomes more difficult for disorders without a definitive treatment. In these cases it is important to emphasize potential screening, avoidance of unnecessary invasive (and expensive) procedures, diet/medication/therapy optimization, and sometimes eligibility for a clinical trial. For example, "If the patient does not have an *FBN1* mutation he can avoid life-long screening echocardiograms" could be a persuasive argument.

As the requested test moves away from single-gene tests to rule in or out a diagnosis toward screening tests, including larger gene panels, microarrays, and exome sequencing, making a convincing case becomes increasingly difficult because the results are hard to predict and therefore hard to connect to a management decision. In these situations, one can try to emphasize the likely high cost of a low-tech diagnostic odyssey, cite literature indicating that these tests are standard-of-care for the clinical situation, or consider the long-term care of the patient. For example, is the patient heading toward major treatment decisions like organ transplantation or tracheostomy, which might be avoided with a clear diagnosis? Is the patient unexpectedly worsening despite (expensive) empiric therapy? Are nongenetic diagnostic maneuvers being considered (e.g., MRI, biopsy, endoscopy) that could be avoided with genetic testing? Clearly describing the patient's clinical evaluation with and without access to genetic testing can be a powerful tool.

Unfortunately, in our experience, arguments such as "the patient will receive improved genetic counseling" or "will be able to make more informed reproductive decisions," while excellent motivations for sending genetic testing, are often not persuasive. If these were convincing, payers would gladly cover testing on deceased individuals to inform the health care of their relatives, which of course they do not. Counseling and reproduction can be mentioned in a letter, but probably not as the primary rationale for testing.

THE HIGH BAR FOR COVERAGE OF GENETIC TESTS

The demand on the part of payers that "results of genetic testing must impact management" is one of the great inconsistencies of the modern medical era. Countless more expensive and more invasive diagnostics (MRIs, CTs, biopsies, exams under anesthesia, endoscopies, etc.) are conducted every minute with a more dubious rationale for management than many genetic tests. The concept that the patient's *diagnosis* is the nexus from which all signs and symptoms are unified, and the kernel from which any future management strategy is formulated, has been the central dogma of medicine for a century.

To think that, at the same moment that medicine finally has the means to diagnose so many more diseases, we turn our backs on this dogma!

Genetic tests are not riskier, more expensive, or more prone to fraud than many other diagnostics in the practice of medicine. Why, then, are genetic tests singled out and a higher bar for coverage applied? We feel there are several possible explanations:

1. Most payers do not understand genetic tests, in large part because the technologies are new and progress rapidly, and have not had time to become comfortable with the complexity in the field.

2. The notion that genetic disease is static and unchangeable—and therefore a diagnosis is of academic value only—is truly outdated yet tragically common.

3. Genetic tests can be ordered by checking a box, making it easier to overtest than more invasive approaches. The accessibility of genetic testing, one of the greatest triumphs of this new technology may be its own enemy.

Yes, the lines between clinical diagnostics and research can be blurry, and assurance of appropriate separations between care and research are needed. Not every genetic test is indicated for a given patient, and high standards of evidence should be applied as in any field. But, in our opinion, to claim that establishing a patient's diagnosis is not important unless there will be an immediate treatment is anachronistic, short-sighted, and inconsistent with the very soul of medicine.

RESOURCES

Molecular diagnostic testing: Alphabet soup with a side of codes (http://www.sciedu.ca/journal/index.php/jha/article/view/8421/5290)

An excellent current review of the molecular diagnostics reimbursement landscape.

NSGC Billing Reimbursement Toolkit (http://www.nsgc.org/members_only/tools/br_index.cfm]

NSGC's Policy and Government Relations department can provide consulting services for a genetic counselor's institution to optimize reimbursement rates. As of September 2010, the fee is $350/hour and the executive office estimated that most institutions would require no more than 1 hour of consultation.

NSGC online course "Learn the 3 C's to Maximize your Service Delivery Model: Coding, Credentialing and Compliance" (http://www.nsgc.org/conferences/CodingCourse2009.cfm)

Defining the role of a genetic counselor as a member of the health care management team; Describing the basics of health care billing; Identifying the complexities of billing for genetic services; Identifying the benefits and limitations of various strategies of billing for genetic services.

MolDx from Palmetto (http://www.palmettogba.com/palmetto/MolDX.nsf/
docsCat/MolDx%20Website~MolDx~Browse%20By%20Topic~Covered%20
Tests?open&Start=1&Count=100&Pg=1&navmenu=Browse^By^Topic||)

Medicare's largest administrative contractor Palmetto, developed MolDx to
evaluate molecular tests and determine whether coverage and reimbursement
will be provided by Medicare.

Evidence and practice guidelines

Several groups curate, evaluate, and synthesize evidence from published
research supporting clinical validity and utility of tests to guide clinicians.

**CDC Office of Public Health Genomics: Guidelines, policies, and rec-
ommendations in genomics** (https://phgkb.cdc.gov/GAPPKB/evidencer.
do?Mysubmit=init&query=&Mysubmit=Search)

The CDC compiles an updated list of guidelines, policies, and recommendations on genomic research and practice, as provided by professional organizations, federal advisory groups, expert panels, and policy groups. The list is
arranged by topics, year of publication, and recommending organization. The
list may not include all relevant recommendations.

**CDC Office of Public Health Genomics: Ranking of genomic tests
and family health history** (https://phgkb.cdc.gov/GAPPKB/topicFinder
.do?Mysubmit=init&query=&Mysubmit=Search)

Provides a 3-tiered classification system based on cumulative evidence[5].

- Tier 1/Green genomic applications have a base of synthesized evidence
that supports implementation in practice.
- Tier 2/Yellow genomic applications have synthesized evidence that is
insufficient to support their implementation in routine practice. Nevertheless, the evidence may be useful for informing selective use strategies
(such as in clinical trials) through individual clinical, or public health
policy, decision-making.
- Tier 3/Red applications either (i) have synthesized evidence that supports
recommendations against or discourages use, or (ii) no relevant synthesized evidence is available.

Eurogentest (www.eurogentest.org)

Based on an initiative of the German Society of Human Genetics, a template
for assessing and describing "indication criteria for genetic testing" was developed, and a series of corresponding guidelines are published in the *European
Journal of Human Genetics* and are now being referred to as Clinical Utility
Gene Cards (CUGCs).

UK Genetic Testing Network (ukgtn.nhs.uk)

Evaluation of new genetic tests that member laboratories wish to provide to NHS patients on a national basis. Examines scientific validity and clinical utility and make recommendations to commissioners. Published as Gene Dossiers.

GeneReviews (genereviews.org)

GeneReviews are expert-authored, peer-reviewed disease descriptions presented in a standardized format and focused on clinically relevant and medically actionable information on the diagnosis, management, and genetic counseling of patients and families with specific inherited conditions.

National Guidelines Clearinghouse (www.guideline.gov)

NGC is a public resource for evidence-based clinical practice guidelines.

REFERENCES

1. Gillis NK, Innocenti F. Evidence required to demonstrate clinical utility of pharmacogenetic testing: the debate continues. *Clin Pharmacol Ther.* 2014;96:655-657.
2. Schork NJ. Personalized medicine: time for one-person trials. *Nature.* 2015;520:609-611.
3. Deverka PA, Dreyfus JC. Clinical integration of next generation sequencing: coverage and reimbursement challenges. *J Law Med Ethics.* 2014;42(suppl 1):22-41.
4. Ubel PA, Abernethy AP, Zafar SY. Full disclosure—out-of-pocket costs as side effects. *N Engl J Med.* 2013;369:1484-1486.
5. Dotson WD, Douglas MP, Kolor K, et al. Prioritizing genomic applications for action by level of evidence: a horizon-scanning method. *Clin Pharmacol Ther.* 2014;95:394-402.
6. Schroeder WS, Demeure MJ and Millis SZ. Molecular diagnostic testing: Alphabet soup with a side of codes. *Journal of Hospital Administration*, 5(2): 2016;p.88-101

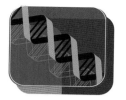

The People in Your Neighborhood

The practice of genetic and genomic medicine spans many professions, and it can be helpful to be familiar with the diverse roles to determine from whom to seek advice and the background and likely skillset of collaborators in patient care. The following is not exhaustive, but covers the most common types of genetics professionals with which one might interact.

MEDICAL GENETICIST

- This professional is almost always an MD (or DO) who has completed training in Medical Genetics and in the United States is board eligible or certified by the American Board of Medical Genetics and Genomics (ABMGG). In the United States, physicians seeking training in Medical Genetics must complete some training in a more general field of medicine. This can range from a full residency and board certification to a single year of general training without board certification. The majority of medical geneticists who see patients in the United States did their general training in Pediatrics, Internal Medicine, or Obstetrics and Gynecology. A smaller number trained in other fields such as Dermatology, Surgery, or Neurology.

- Some physicians who complete training in Medical Genetics are pathologists and are critical for the implementation and interpretation of genetic laboratory tests.

- Other countries have different training models for Genetics, such as an inclusive program where pediatric, adult, and obstetric medicine are combined into the same program for all geneticists.

- Among physician medical geneticists, there is a substantial degree of subspecialization. Some geneticists see a broad range of ages and conditions (sometimes referred to as "General Genetics"). Others only see adult conditions (cardiovascular disease, cancer, neurodegeneration). Other common specialties involve metabolic/biochemical disease, neurologic disease, autism, skeletal dysplasia, prenatal genetics and maternal and fetal medicine, or diseases confined to one organ system (eye, skin, etc.). Due to the vastness of genetic knowledge, specialization is becoming more common, with each physician practicing in some subset of the above fields. It is very important to identify the proper specialist for any patient referral: no two geneticists are alike!

NONGENETICIST SPECIALIST PHYSICIANS

- More and more, the application of genomic medicine is taking place under the care of physicians who do not have formal training in Medical Genetics but have experience diagnosing and treating inherited conditions unique to their specialty, which can span the full breadth of medicine and surgery. Not uncommonly, these specialists have more expertise in a particular condition than a general geneticist. An example might be a dermatologist who specializes in inherited skin conditions. Consulting a medical geneticist for any disease involving DNA is probably not feasible, but excellent collaboration among all specialists is a worthy goal to be sure that tests are sent and interpreted appropriately and that pre- and post-test counseling is adequate. Team medicine is certainly an important trend that without question will involve genetic and genomic medicine.

GENETIC COUNSELOR

- Genetic counselors are nonphysician specialists who have extensive training in the mechanisms of inheritance, genetic diseases, and diagnostics, often with a focus on translating this knowledge into excellent communication with patients. Genetic and genomic medicine require the assimilation of complex patient information, data from literature, and the synthesis, communication of tests, diagnoses, and risks, and many administrative tasks navigating the medical system. Genetic counselors are trained in all these areas, but in reality, the roles of genetic counselors vary widely across genetics practices.

- In the United States, genetic counselors cannot prescribe medications or perform other duties that are reserved for physicians. Nevertheless, in some states genetic counselors can bill for time spent with patients and can work more or less autonomously for patients that do not require medications or other physician services. In others they must work under a licensed physician, and in either case may be able to act in a capacity akin to that of a nurse practitioner or physician's assistant. In some practices all patients see a counselor and a physician. In others, patients may see one, the other, or both depending on the clinical need.

- Recently, diagnostic laboratories have been hiring genetic counselors to provide support to practitioners ordering tests, to guide test development, to perform marketing and research, and to conduct the still largely manual task of variant interpretation. This will likely continue to be an active area of employment growth.

- Like physician geneticists, genetic counselors often have a field (or few fields) of expertise, covering the same range of conditions and patient populations.

LABORATORY DIRECTORS

- Any diagnostic laboratory (biochemical, cytogenetics, sequencing, etc.) requires a laboratory director. The director can be an MD or a PhD who has completed laboratory training under the ABMGG (in the United States), which oversees both clinical and laboratory certifications.

- Lab directors are critical to test design and development, quality assurance, regulatory oversight, technological innovation, test interpretation, and communicating with ordering physicians. It is usually possible (and desirable) to talk to the laboratory director with questions about a test. At some labs, genetic counselors or laboratory genetics trainees may be the first-line providers of test information, depending on the question.

RESOURCES

American Board of Medical Genetics and Genomics (http://www.abmgg .org/pages/searchmem.shtml)

On this page one can search for a geneticist in the United States by name or by city/state and by specialty.

National Society of Genetic Counselors (NSGC.org)

Professional association of genetic counselors. Website includes educational resources and tools to help locate a genetic counselor.

Informed DNA (Informeddna.com)

Independent network of genetic counselors.

NCI Cancer Genetics Services Directory (cancer.gov/cancertopics/genetics/ directory)

This directory lists professionals who provide services related to cancer genetics (cancer risk assessment, genetic counseling, genetic susceptibility testing, and others).

GeneTests Clinical Directory (genetests.org)

A medical genetics information resource.

Crosscutting Ethical Issues

Eugenics, and the fear thereof, are common themes in ethical discussions of genomic technologies during reproduction that many are not quite proficient at discussing. Leaving aside concerns about creating super-people, let us simply consider the application of genetics to bona fide diseases. Preventing lethal infections is hardly controversial, and no one advocates against vaccination on the grounds that people with Pertussis represent an important facet of humanity we would be poorer without, and few believe we should "leave nature alone" and accept serious infections. One might therefore call a disease a disease, regardless of the cause, and would say a distinction between infectious and inherited disease is a false dichotomy. But perhaps because our genes make us who we are, selecting against certain genes, no matter how cruel the phenotype, gives many the sensation that humanity is meddling where it shouldn't with feelings that are not aroused by other fields of medicine. Are we changing who we are rather than how the outside world affects us? The greatest challenge of the coming genomics era, when we can sequence and even change our genes with ease, will be for society and individuals to mature in our understanding of basic ideas such as self, family, choice, and worth as we wield more control of our fundamental biology that until now was in the hands of evolution, chance, and the Divine.

Either way, it is difficult not to admit that the broad demand for genetic screening for inherited/genetic diseases implies that many societies value health over disability, whether intrinsic (i.e., genetic) or extrinsic. Recognizing and confessing our own biases, even as medicine churns out newer and better screening tests, is essential for any practitioner to provide sensitive and balanced care and counseling for patients regarding inherited disease.

Inevitably, as payers increasingly cover expanded carrier screening, and have no choice but to cover increasingly available (and very expensive) therapies for children with genetic diseases, some payers will attempt to control costs by offering to cover PGD completely to prevent the birth of sick and expensive children. This would be tremendously empowering for families that could not otherwise afford to have a healthy child, but would also greatly increase the frequency with which embryos were actively decided to be unfit to be implanted or born. Such selection is completely legal and available today to those who can pay for it, but increased availability (and possibly public funding) are at least psychologically more salient for a society and are likely to stir more heated discussion and disagreement.

Diseases that kill in the first days of life are less controversial as targets of carrier screening, and likewise eye color is not (to our knowledge) a trait on which any reputable reproductive specialist would agree to base the selection of an embryo. There are, however, gray zones of diseases that are harder to categorize. Is a heightened risk of Alzheimer disease reason to select against an embryo? Is a disease that is serious in 2% of cases, but manageable in the other 98% a good reason? Who decides? We are not waiting for any new technologies to make these questions relevant today; rather, it is our opinion that it is primarily the cost barrier to PGD and IVF that keeps these questions off the radar, a situation that will not last forever.

GENETIC TESTING OF MINORS

A fundamental principle of medical ethics is patient autonomy. Whenever possible, patients should be permitted to make informed decisions as to their health care, rather than have decisions forced upon them by the medical establishment, or even their own parents. Minors present a challenge because, legally, they cannot consent to medical tests or procedures. Medicine infers consent (or seeks assent), or allows the parents to act in the best interest of a child, when illness strikes a minor. But that child will one day be an adult, and any permanent decisions made in childhood by definition deprive the adult of his or her autonomy. This is why we generally do not encourage elective cosmetic surgery, permit sterilization, or perform gender reassignment surgery on minors.

The same concept holds true for genetic testing. Every adult has a right to decline to know information about his or her genetic risks, and testing that adult when they are still a minor impinges on that right. For example, a woman with a family history of breast cancer may prefer not to undergo genetic testing to clarify her personal risk. How dare we force that knowledge on her by testing her as a child!

Put bluntly, genetic or genomic testing on a minor should not be performed unless the minor is symptomatic and in need of a diagnosis, or the test is specifically targeted to diseases that present in childhood (like newborn screening). Infrequently, testing of minors is appropriate to clarify genetic test results in a family member. This challenge will only grow as newer genetic tests focus on analyzing many (or all) genes at once. Performing genome-wide tests and then intentionally releasing the information piecemeal as the patient ages seems paternalistic and anachronistic, and yet may be the most efficient and ethical way to proceed. Patient buy-in, where consumers and parents understand and respect the benefits and risks of genetic knowledge across one's lifespan, will play a key role in ensuring the ethical deployment of genomic technologies.

ETHICS OF PRENATAL SCREENING

Probably the major ethical conundrum with prenatal testing, at least until in utero therapies exist for more than a handful of disorders, is the fact that generally the only "intervention" available when a disease is detected is termination of the pregnancy. Few topics are as divisive and controversial as abortion, and increased prenatal screening may increase the number of pregnancies that are terminated when disease is detected. Whatever one's opinion is toward abortion, most would agree that helping families to have healthy children while reducing the frequency with which a woman is faced with the decision to have an abortion would be desirable. Several approaches, some easier than others, can accomplish this goal.

First, the sensitivity and specificity of any prenatal screen must be well understood by the practitioner. Noninvasive prenatal screening, while a substantial advancement beyond traditional quad screening, is still not as definitive as amniocentesis. Appropriately tailoring screening to the risks and wishes of each family may reduce unanticipated decisions about continuing a pregnancy. More detailed tests such as microarrays, when applied to a fetus, may reveal a variant of unknown significance, or one with a variable phenotype, and every effort must be made to provide the family with accurate, unbiased information and not sensationalize a finding beyond the best available evidence. Most importantly, difficult decisions can be mitigated by educating patients about any genetic testing *before* it is sent.

UNEQUAL ACCESS AND THE COST OF HEALTH CARE

New technologies, particularly expensive new technologies, are met with resistance from health care payers for obvious reasons. Beyond the issue of payments, access simply spreads slower in rural regions with fewer specialists and to individuals of lower socioeconomic status for a host of other complex reasons. As was discussed in Chapter 5, genomic medicine has joined a long list of other health care services to which individuals around the world and even in the same country have grossly unequal access. *TIME* magazine (March 19, 2015 "The Cancer Gap") covered the stark difference in cancer care received by women based mostly on location and insurance, for example.

Beyond simple fairness, societies run the risk of changing genetic diseases from equalizers based on our common humanity into just another marker of wealth, much as infectious disease burden reflects income today (think of tuberculosis). Just a few years ago, the wealthiest couple had the same risk of having a child with a rare recessive disease as a poor couple. Today, with rapidly advancing preconception and prenatal screening, many genetic diseases are avoidable to those with resources. The same can be said of adult-onset disease, cancer, and pharmacogenomics.

A common refrain during genetic counseling sessions is an emphasis on humanity's helplessness to control the genes we inherit and pass on. A grieving couple would typically be comforted that there was no way they could have known they both carried the same ultrarare lethal genetic disease, and no way they could have controlled the alleles they transmitted to their ill-fated child. Today, for many diseases, these words of comfort are increasingly untrue. Yes, long-term studies of many screening modalities are lacking, as are cost-effectiveness analyses, but no one seriously doubts that in many fields of medicine genetic screening will become the rule in short order. Perhaps, with this impending revolution, societies will break with tradition and make sure no one is left behind.

WHO OWNS YOUR GENOME?

This topic primarily arises in discussions of direct-to-consumer genetic testing, and much has been written on the topic. To paraphrase Robert Nussbaum, a pioneer in human genetics, the question is not unlike that posed during the Protestant Reformation in Europe: do people require an intermediary between themselves and their genomes, or can they have a direct relationship? On one hand, one's DNA is unique and personal, and it seems logical to assert ownership and control over it. On the other hand, understanding sequencing results is complex and analogous to other types of tests like MRIs or echocardiograms, which can only be obtained through a physician's order and interpretation.

Practically, this question could be answered in different ways. In the United States, the Food and Drug Administration (FDA) is considering regulating genetic testing much more broadly (see Appendix 7), and this could restrict or slow progress in direct-to-consumer testing. There is certainly some consumer demand for direct-to-consumer testing, but the fraction of the population that is interested in this beyond early adopters will depend on the utility of testing, cost, and accessibility through more traditional avenues (i.e., the health care system). If medical professionals are able to provide sufficiently efficient access to clinically appropriate genetic testing then direct-to-consumer testing may be less relevant.

Society will certainly evolve in its understanding of the role of genetic testing. Success stories of improved health and empowerment will spur testing, while confusion and public expressions of regret will slow it. Genetics and its terminology will enter high school curricula and the popular vernacular. Software may partially replace more basic facets of genetic counseling, allowing individuals to safely navigate their genomes with a clearer understanding of what information they seek or wish to avoid. Electronic health records will be able to import genomic data and usefully integrate it into the medical history, drug allergies/contraindications, and health screening. Thus, the question of genome ownership will become at once more complex and less relevant as the evidence of utility of genomic testing and ease of access increase with time.

PRIVACY (GINA)

Privacy concerns have become pervasive in our digital society and genomics has not been spared. Privacy issues in genomics can roughly be divided into concerns about information being leaked to those who have no business seeing it (hackers) and to those with some legitimacy but dubious intentions (insurers, the government, employers, etc.). The former is predominantly a technological matter, though it bears mention that the surest way to keep information private is not to generate it in the first place.

In the United States, some protection is offered by GINA, the Genetic Information Non-discrimination Act of 2008. It prevents genetic information from being used to determine health insurance coverage or rates and for matters related to employment. It does *not* provide protection for life, disability, or long-term care insurance. Discussing how genetic information might be used is an important part of consenting to genetic tests, especially when one is screening rather than seeking a diagnosis, since in the latter case the disease itself likely impacts insurance eligibility more than any test result might.

INCIDENTAL/SECONDARY FINDINGS ON WHOLE-EXOME/WHOLE-GENOME SEQUENCING

Nothing pains a geneticist more than hearing a patient say, "I wish I'd never had this test." Almost universally such regret comes from a test whose scope the patient did not fully appreciate, usually due to inadequate pretest counseling. Other times, inappropriate tests (e.g., MTHFR, ApoE4) are sent due to a mistaken belief about their diagnostic/prognostic value.

Our genomes are (at least for the moment) immutable, and thus genetic test results are forever (literally, if the patient has children). Ordering physicians and other providers have an obligation to be sure that patients understand what is being sent, that some tests return results unrelated to the purpose of the test (incidental findings or secondary findings), and that everyone has genetic variation that may or may not be interpretable in terms of their health.

Not all unexpected findings are without value, however. The ACMG has issued a statement on reporting of incidental findings from genome-scale sequencing tests (such as whole-genome or whole-exome sequencing). Its consensus is that, though ironclad evidence of clinical utility from reporting incidental findings is lacking, some carefully selected genes would be clinically actionable in most individuals and warrant reporting when pathogenic variants are detected. This is not the same as recommending universal screening of healthy individuals for these disorders.

The ACMG's recommendations for reporting incidental findings can be summarized as follows:

- Laboratories should actively search for pathogenic variants in the recommended gene list.

- Variants of uncertain significance should not be reported (unless they may relate to the primary phenotype for which the test was sent).

- The depth-of-coverage of genes on the recommended list need not meet a certain standard.

- An absence of incidental findings should not be construed as having definitively ruled out a disease caused by genes on the recommended list.
- Patients can opt out of receiving incidental findings. Importantly, the ACMG struggled with this concept. The ACMG understandably felt that withholding actionable health information was ethically questionable. Indeed, patients undergoing many other types of tests (e.g., brain MRI) do not have the choice to withhold certain results selectively. True, the patient may have opted out of receiving incidental genetic findings, but the ACMG questioned the feasibility of adequately counseling for all the different clinical scenarios represented by the recommended gene list. Most clinical geneticists discourage opting out but discuss the option out of respect for the patient's autonomy.
- It is acceptable to report the same incidental findings in a minor even for adult-onset conditions because the findings were likely inherited and may be actionable for the parents. In the future, when adults have ready access to overlapping testing targeted at actionable genes, it would be more appropriate to withhold adult-onset results in minors because the parents could easily obtain this information for themselves.
- Pre- and post-test counseling remain critical.
- More data on patient preferences, frequency of incidental findings, improved knowledge of disease penetrance, availability of better sequencing and bioinformatics systems, and other progress in genomics will likely modify many of these recommendations. The concept itself of incidental findings may be entirely transient, as genome-scale testing becomes more and more routine earlier and earlier in life and systems are developed to incorporate all findings into health care maintenance.

RESOURCE

ACMG Recommendations for Reporting of Incidental Findings (https://www .acmg.net/docs/ACMG_Releases_Highly-Anticipated_Recommendations _on_Incidental_Findings_in_Clinical_Exome_and_Genome_Sequencing.pdf)

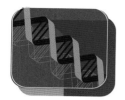

Horizons in Genomic Medicine

GENE EDITING

The possibility of gene editing (actually physically fixing a disease-causing mutation) in an embryo or human tissue is quickly becoming a reality. Several different technologies permit gene editing, but currently the most promising is based on CRISPR/Cas9. The Cas9 enzyme is part of a rudimentary bacterial immune system that binds to a guide RNA, finds the complementary DNA sequence, and cuts it. Bacteria use the CRISPR system to defend themselves against invading viruses, but the same technology can be harnessed to make a cut almost anywhere in the human genome. Additional DNA can then be added to replace the DNA around the cut site. Any alteration in an embryo or in a germ cell (predecessor to an egg or sperm) would be passed on indefinitely in future generations. This technology is not yet highly efficient, but progress has been stunning and major advancements are inevitable.

For the purpose of preventing recessive disease, when compared with traditional PGD, this approach does not offer any benefit because if multiple embryos are formed with traditional PGD (see Chapter 1), statistically some of them will not be affected and can be implanted. Gene editing offers the possibility of creating, repairing, and implanting only one embryo, which might be more palatable to parents who consider life to begin at conception and would not consider fertilizing several eggs and discarding some. Gene editing would also enhance selection against multiple conditions simultaneously because one would not need to find the improbable embryo that was free of all the traits under consideration, but rather could select the embryo with the fewest conditions and repair the rest.

CRISPR technology could be used to treat a wide variety of diseases and is an area of breakneck research. Some approaches seek to edit cancer cells, others alter the immune system, and some insert missing genes into organs such as the liver or retina. The endless possibilities have certainly not been fully studied to date and this or related technologies are likely to stay at the forefront of biomedicine for years to come.

The most ethically concerning use of CRISPR technology would be the editing of an embryo to possess alleles or genes not present in either parent. Such technology is already available, and if or how such genetic manipulation will be regulated is difficult to predict. Society will need to come to grips with the breakdown of the immutability of the genome and place appropriate safeguards that prevent harm while permitting the treatment of disease.

MITOCHONDRIAL TRANSFER (3-PARENT BABIES)

Another recent reproductive technology offers hope to mothers with mutations in their mitochondrial DNA. All of a child's mitochondrial DNA is inherited from the mother, so a woman with a mutation in the mitochondrial DNA in her eggs could pass this disease to 100% of her biological children.

Avoiding this seemingly certain fate requires that a mother's egg be fertilized, but then the new nucleus is transferred to another woman's egg. What results is the woman's biological child, but with a third person's mitochondrial DNA (much less than 1% of the total DNA in the cell). Few children have been born as a result of this technique, and thus precise data on this procedure's safety are lacking, but compared to a near-certain probability of a mitochondrial disease, this approach may be of significant benefit for women with defined mitochondrial disorders.

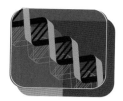

Useful Links for Genomic Medicine

Genetic testing and diagnostics
www.nextgxdx.com/
www.genetests.org/

Genome browsers
genome.ucsc.edu/
www.ensembl.org/

Disease information
omim.org/
www.rarechromo.org/
www.ncbi.nlm.nih.gov/books/NBK1116/
elementsofmorphology.nih.gov/

Patient-centered disease information
www.umdf.org/
ghr.nlm.nih.gov/
www.rarechromo.org/
www.babysfirsttest.org/

Newborn screening
www.babysfirsttest.org/
www.newbornscreening.info/
genes-r-us.uthscsa.edu/

Advocacy and support
www.raregenomics.org/
www.mitoaction.org/
www.umdf.org/
www.acmg.net/
everylifefoundation.org/
globalgenes.org/
www.genome.gov/
www.acmg.net/ACMG/Advocacy/ACMG/Advocacy/Advocacy.aspx?hkey
=759c3556-90cb-42a7-ba8d-af07742bf941

Trisomy 21 advocacy and support
www.ndsccenter.org/
www.ndss.org/

Variant databases and support

genematcher.org/
www.ncbi.nlm.nih.gov/clinvar/intro/
cancer.sanger.ac.uk/cosmic
exac.broadinstitute.org/
www.1000genomes.org/
dgv.tcag.ca/dgv/app/home

Physician/practitioner education and support

geneticsinprimarycare.aap.org/
genes-r-us.uthscsa.edu/resources/genetics/primary_care.htm
www.geneticmetabolic.com/
newbornscreeningeducation.org/
www.acmg.net/ACMG/Publications/Practice_Guidelines/ACMG/Publications/
Practice_Guidelines.aspx
g-2-c-2.org/
www.pathologylearning.org/trig/resources

Rare disease search engines: Note that these search engines cannot replace sound clinical experience and should be used only to supplement more traditional diagnostic approaches.

findzebra.compute.dtu.dk/
omim.org/
www.simulconsult.com/

Nutrition and dietary

dsld.nlm.nih.gov/dsld/

Metabolic disease

www.geneticmetabolic.com/
www.genome.gov/27551373

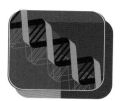

Index

Note: Page numbers with a *t* indicate a table. Page numbers with an *f* indicate a figure.